Managing Cardiovascular Risk In Elective Total Joint Arthroplasty

Eric E. Harrison • Nghia H. Ho
Editors

Managing Cardiovascular Risk In Elective Total Joint Arthroplasty

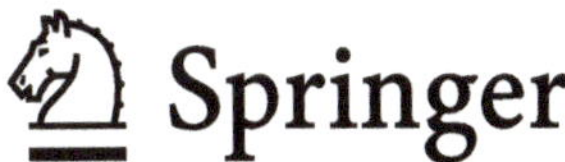

Editors
Eric E. Harrison
Morsani College of Medicine
University of South Florida
Tampa, FL, USA

Nghia H. Ho
Harrison Cardiovascular Clinic
Tampa, FL, USA

ISBN 978-3-031-26417-7 ISBN 978-3-031-26415-3 (eBook)
https://doi.org/10.1007/978-3-031-26415-3

This Springer imprint is published by the registered company Springer Nature Switzerland AG
The registered company address is: Gewerbestrasse 11, 6330 Cham, Switzerland

This book is dedicated to the active and retired National Football League players who are competitive and high performance athletes that entertain us in the Fall and Winter of every year. The retired players have a high profile for orthopedic and cardiac risk at a younger age. It is our goal to foresee these problems and prevent them, which is the goal of this book.

– Eric E. Harrison, MD

Foreword

The only thing I hated more than losing a game when I was the owner of the San Francisco 49ers was losing a player to injury. All these men were like sons and brothers to me. Their significant others were like sisters and daughters.

When the story of the 49ers is told, it often begins with the five Super Bowl Championships we won during the 1980s and 1990s. But it's really a story about family.

When one of my players became injured, it was like watching a member of my family in pain.

I used to leave the game and meet them in the locker room or ride in the ambulance with them to the hospital.

I'll never forget the worst injury I ever witnessed was when one of our best players, defensive tackle Bryant Young, went down during a Monday Night Football game against the New York Giants. My heart dropped out of my chest because he was like the Rock Gibraltar. He was injured by friendly fire. Teammate Ken Norton inadvertently slammed his helmet into Young's shin while trying to make a tackle and the bones in his leg shattered.

His pregnant wife, Kristin, held one hand and I held the other during the 25-mile trip to Stanford Hospital. I grabbed a pair of scissors and began cutting off his jersey. Paramedics were struggling to put the intravenous needle in Young's arm, so I yelled, "Pull this damn ambulance over and get the IV started."

Remarkably, after 9 months of rehab, Young returned to the field and had 9.5 sacks the following season.

But the sense of responsibility I felt toward Young, and all our 49ers family, has endured long after their playing days ended. So has their need to overcome and recover from so many debilitating injuries that worsen after retirement from football.

The physical toll the game takes on them makes them more susceptible to long-term health challenges. Many studies have shown that professional football players have higher risk factors and a much greater incidence of cardiac episodes than the general population after their playing days are over.

I've never stopped caring for these men, and when I recently needed a hip replacement, I was introduced to an innovative procedure in cardiac care pioneered by Dr. Eric E. Harrison, M.D.

Utilizing advanced 3D imaging technology, Dr. Harrison is able to show who is considered safe to undergo orthopedic surgery and who is at risk to have a cardiac event and then proactively treat people that are high risk before their orthopedic surgery. Many hip and knee replacement patients seem to have postoperative cardiac problems and this technology can predict it.

This procedure isn't mainstream yet, but it's gaining momentum and should become part of the normal preoperative process, especially for people at risk who have hypertension, family heart disease, high cholesterol, and obesity, like many current and retired NFL players do.

Using this 3D CT-based planning, Dr. Harrison is able to control the surgery with data obtained from the scan, which always makes for cleaner and safer outcomes.

Think of it as a different way of looking at the heart. Rather than catheterization, which injects dye into the arteries to detect if there is blockage, this tells surgeons whether the plaque is safe or soft, whether it has a chance to rupture and cause a heart attack.

It gave me great comfort to know I had very minimal risk of a heart attack before I underwent my hip replacement surgery in 2020.

I strongly encourage and support Dr. Harrison's effort to radically change cardio-orthopedics. I'm confident that his innovative approach will help save the lives of countless patients and hopefully lead to healthier lives for members of not just our 49ers family, but your loved ones as well.

Edward J. DeBartolo Jr. is a successful businessman, real estate investor and developer, Hall of Fame sports owner, and passionate supporter of philanthropic causes related to education, healthcare, poverty, animals, sports, and religious institutions. A graduate of the University of Notre Dame, Mr. DeBartolo is the chief executive officer of DeBartolo Holdings, LLC, which manages the diversified businesses and strategic investments of the DeBartolo family, including real estate and sports. He is best known as the legendary owner of the San Francisco 49ers who won 5 Super Bowl Championships and 12 division titles during his 23-year ownership and management of the team. Affectionately called "Mr. D" by his players, he is widely regarded as one of the most compassionate owners in NFL history and was inducted into the Pro Football Hall of Fame in 2016. Mr. DeBartolo resides in Tampa, Fla., with his wife Candy. They have three daughters, Lisa Marie, Tiffanie Lynne, and Nicole Anne, and three grandsons, Asher, Milo, and Jasper.

San Francisco, CA, USA — Edward J. DeBartolo Jr

Preface

I'm here to tell you today about something we started a long time ago, about 2016 called cardio-orthopedics. So we're professionals at bridging silos. We have the DeBartolo Society for bridging medical silos, the parent company of these other companies: cardio-oncology which is a bridge of two silos. We brought these two things together very successfully. It was important because women with cancer of the breast were getting congestive heart failure and 18% were dying, and we figured out how to spot that and prevent it. We were successful 9 years ago at doing that and developing that into a whole regimen, thanks to Steve Casselli, and thanks to Dan Lenihan, MD.

My job was to consider something that I'd seen among patients that was worrying me. With 5000 patients in our practice and a curated patient database, I became worried about patients that had orthopedic problems and also cardiac problems. Let me give you an example. We had a great preacher that I really liked a lot. He's had some bypass surgery and some stents. We took good care of him. His cardiac status was great. Then, he's scheduled for hip surgery. He went into Memorial Hospital. He's going to get his surgery. The doctors who were responsible for him was an orthopedist who was an older orthopedist. He had a good anesthesiologist, I believe. Our preacher friend had the surgery. I went to the hospital to see him after the surgery. He was in shock. It was 7:00 pm. Anesthesiologist was gone. The orthopedist was gone. There was a chart with no notes. I had to figure out what to do with this gentleman: why is he in shock? I had to go get the echo machine going and doing the EKG… all these things we had to do, he's dying, and I don't know why. He's not in septic shock. I found that he's bleeding, and he's been bleeding since the surgery. He was bleeding in the OR. Apparently, there was a problem regulating his drugs, or he had been on Plavix and aspirin. I don't know when they stopped them or how long they stopped them, but now they had stopped them and yet he's still bleeding. He didn't survive that.

I felt terrible about that. I started looking at our database. I curated patients and tried to figure out what it is that happens to these people. Some of them are bundled—CMS bundles the patients and their payment into $2530; this is a lump sum payment. If anything goes wrong, you have to give some of that back. Maybe you would say the orthopedist in the hospital has skin in the game. That's pretty important. Bundled patients. So I called these patients who were getting in trouble who were prolonged in the hospital or we were re-admitting with problems. I called them "Bundle Busters." I wanted to find out about the Bundle Busters and what went wrong with them, and why. So I looked through the list. I found that with patients having knee surgery or hip surgery all had problems with heart attacks. You had to get a stent. You had a bleeding. You had pulmonary embolus. You got worse because you're getting medicines that suppress your breathing. Which were pain medicines? All these things were very, very complicated. They stopped your anti-coagulation before surgery a week before and you came in and had a stroke. I mean, these are very, very complicated things, and so I said, "well, what's wrong?" and I tried to find things I could change: maybe I need to have a different hospital. So I sent the patient to a different hospital. I said well, maybe I need to have a different operating room, so I sent them to a different operating room. Maybe I need to have a different surgeon and so we went through all that stuff. And I said, you know? I think what I really need is a different cardiologist; I was the problem! I'm blaming myself. Why am I blaming myself? Well, I'm using traditional medical treatment on these patients, and for some reason, they're not meeting what my expectations were. And so I decided, after having looked at the database, that maybe if I go forward, maybe I'd do something different. Maybe if we do a preop evaluation that's more than just running an EKG, more than just doing an echocardiogram and saying it's OK. Maybe I need to do a full assessment and then do a cardiac CT—actually look at the heart. I get the list of medications that they are on. I do an echocardiogram. And if I think there're episodes of atrial fibrillation, perhaps I should do a recording of their heartbeat for 3 or 4 days, or maybe a week and see if they're having PVCs or atrial fibrillation. I saw that hypertension was very common. I saw that some of them had dilated aortas. Some people had low ejection fractions. Some people had paroxysmal atrial fibrillation. Some people were on blood thinners. Some people had pulmonary embolus, and they were present before the surgery on the CT scan. Some people had had a previous stroke. What I discovered is that these were a very complicated group of patients that we need to have a better understanding than we do, especially with people over 65.

After this realization, a gentleman came along. He was a nice gentleman who's 68 years old and had pericarditis 15 years ago, had atrial fibrillation at that time, and then he had an endoscopy recently. So he came over to see me. I told him we're going to do this CT scan and we're going to do the echo. And then we're going to see if there's anything else wrong. So we did the CT scan and we found a lesion. And we can show you that lesion that I was worried about with our AI software. I was worried about it because it was a set up to having a severe problem. You might say, we would show you how to predict a heart attack. This book will show you what we found and why that became important. We found that he (our patient) had a blockage in his coronary, which was about 70%, but more important than that was there's an ulcer in the middle of this blockage. How is this going to be a problem? Well, you probably don't know, but I do! Because 27 years ago, I had a patient that had a similar lesion demonstrated from a cardiac cath. I'd seen that and she was going to have surgery on her right hip. She was in surgery and I bought the echo machine in and I'm looking at her right atrium and the right ventricle and I see this bone powder come rushing in. It's like a snowstorm! It's like taking a globe at Christmastime, and shaking it up and seeing the snow surround frosty the snowman. All this stuff came in and was bone powder. And microscopically you could tell that it had fibrin on both ends, and it was a powerful platelet activator, and so if that activates the platelets, within 24 h on this patient, then that bone powder with platelet activation is going to deposit itself in this plaque ulcer and it's going to occlude the vessel. So we predicted that was going to happen to the patient. So, in preparation we got a nurse navigator to see him. Canceled his surgery where it was going to be at a big hospital with 15 patients getting their hips done and scheduled him for his hip in a local hospital. He goes to Memorial Hospital and has the hip surgery. After the surgery, he is sent home. Then, the next day while sitting at home drinking a cup of coffee, he started having severe chest pain. He knew he would have this episode based on what I "predicted." So he called his daughter back to pick him up. He called the nurse navigator at the hospital and said, "I'm having chest pain" and they rushed him over, did a cardiac cath, found the clot in there and put a stent in. Saved his life. Saved $20,000. Then he went home in just a couple of days and he was fine.

So we said, "Look, we could predict these patients can have a heart attack. Not only that, but we can predict they can have many problems, including atrial fibrillation, dilated left ventricle or aneurysm, pulmonary emboli coronary artery disease." All these things are the pieces of the puzzle. And these pieces of the puzzle are very, very important: hypertension, LVH—we can monitor their heart for 24 h, detect if they are going to have atrial fibrillation, they have strokes, they have aortic stenosis, they have an aortic aneurysm, pulmonary emboli, they're at risk of having a heart attack. All these things, and that's why one out of seven patients over age 65 get troponin elevations, which is a cardiac marker that may show cardiac injury but may not be predictive of a heart attack. We've got patients over 65 going to surgery and we've got to check them. So we aligned ourselves with Florida Orthopaedic Institute, who decided they were going to send their patients to me and they would pick about 30%. They would be over 70 for sure. Some over 65. They would be at high risk. We would see about 500 of them. We would show them that what is wrong with them is predictable. It is predictable. It's not something that just happens randomly. It is predictable. With these pieces of the puzzle, we actually came up with our own score called the OSCARS score. The OSCARS score is something that is a number telling you what their risk is, but it's also a number that, if we have 30 days to treat, we can reduce their number before they go to surgery and they can go to surgery and have outpatient surgery. And no complications, so that's what our goal was and that's what we achieved. And that was the start of cardio-orthopedics.

So we think that this is something we can apply in other hospitals and we think it's very important to get away from what we did in the past, which is only a simple EKG and you go to surgery or a simple echo and you go to surgery. That 30% of these patients are at high risk and we can evaluate what's wrong with them? Contain it, control it. 75% have hypertension, 11% have paroxysmal atrial fibrillation, about

20% have chronic and paroxysmal atrial fibrillation. A smaller percentage are at risk of having a heart attack. That was the formation of cardio-orthopedics. I hope to teach you more about this. We're going to continue to do the work we've done since 2016. Medicine is very slow to change.

Tampa, FL, USA Eric E. Harrison

Contents

1 Preface

Eric E. Harrison

Abstract

This chapter introduces by way of case review, anecdotal evidence and evidence-based experience, the need for closer cooperation between orthopedics and cardiology, particularly in relation to total joint arthroplasty (TJA). The use of computerized axial tomography scans (CT scans) is recommended as a preoperative diagnostic tool along with echocardiography. The rationale for the use of noninvasive cardiac imaging is explained, and the necessity for a comprehensive workup vis-a-vis cardio-orthopedics is justified by our observational comparison readmission rate before and after the institution of cardiac imaging prior to surgery.

Keywords

Cardio-orthopedics · Total joint arthroplasty (TJA) · Preoperative evaluation · Cardiac risk of TJA · Perioperative risk assessment

E. E. Harrison (✉)
Board Chair International Cardio-Oncology Society,
ICOS CEO PrivaCors Inc. Cardio-Orthopaedics®, Tampa, FL, USA

Morsani College of Medicine, University of South Florida, Tampa, FL, USA

Joint Special Operations University, MacDill Air Force Base, Tampa, FL, USA

E. E. Harrison, N. H. Ho (eds.), *Managing Cardiovascular Risk In Elective Total Joint Arthroplasty*, https://doi.org/10.1007/978-3-031-26415-3_1

Learning Objectives

Patients over the age of 65 with a history of heart disease have frequent post-TJA cardiac complications that were not predictable by our cardiac historical risk models. A new model of cardiac imaging has evolved replacing stress tests and diagnostic cath with coronary CTA and complex cardiovascular ultrasound allowing for opportunities to build new risk models based on anatomy rather than history. Silos of medicine inhibit collaboration and advances. Cardio-oncology was created to bridge two important silos with great success. In orthopedics, our employing anatomical models allowed for a whole new recognition of underlying heart disease for the development of predictive models of events that were not foreseeable. This has evolved over time into a new silo bridge creating cardio-orthopedics, a way to bring together the specialists to assess cardiac risk and control it.

You are asking yourself why is a cardiologist writing about orthopedics and why combine cardiology with orthopedics? Ten years ago, I would have asked the same thing. I have a cardiology clinical practice in Tampa, Florida, where I have been a cardiologist for 45 years. The clinic has a patient base of about 5000 people. Many have been my patients for over 30 years where I'm the family cardiologist and have a close personal relationship with all of them since they enrolled in my practice prior cardiology becoming industrialized by the implementation of Electronic Medical Records (EMR), insurers controlling patients by preauthorization of their medications and procedures, cardiology practices being acquired by hospitals and other organizations whereby timed patient visits based on Relative Value Units (RVUs), and computer keyboards detract from patient–physician relationships.

You will find this book is very case oriented because these cases not only illustrate careful practice but also serve as awakening examples that may suggest new research ideas and hypotheses.

For example, a 60-year-old lady was scheduled for a total hip arthroplasty (THA) but had a known asymptomatic significant proximal 70% left anterior descending lesion on cardiac catheterization which had been done a year before. Out of concern of heart ischemia during surgery, the decision was made to do an intraoperative transesophageal echocardiography (TEE) during the THA in order to watch the anterior wall, apex, and IV septum during the surgery. If regional wall motion changes were observed, the action would be to start a nitroglycerine drip to attenuate the ischemia. All was going well until during the rongeuring of the femoral head by the surgeon, a sudden rush of contrast-like material swirled into the right atrium, right ventricle, and pulmonary arteries not unlike one sees with echo contrast studies. The surgeon was so taken aback by this appearance that he commanded me to turn off the echo machine. The patient did well, and this was merely an incidental finding. But this was my first introduction to the convergence of the two specialties.

Over time my aging cardiac patients frequently needed surgical clearance for total joint arthroplasty. My statements of risk at first were based on the Goldman Criteria, then the Modified Goldman Criteria which was a summation of mostly historical cardiac information. The risk estimation seemed adequate but patients with low risk had unanticipated cardiac problems which did not seem to conform to my calculated risk. One gentleman in his late 70s, who had coronary stents with aspirin on hold for 10 days and clopidogrel for 5 days, did poorly and came out of surgery in shock from continued bleeding into his hip. Another lady in her 80s with hypertension had THA developed postoperative angina and was stented. A gentleman with a history of paroxysmal atrial fibrillation (PAF)) on medical therapy missed his anti-arrhythmic medication dose and was pushed into the ICU with AF with rapid ventricular response (RVR) after TKA. A male in his 70s with prior remote Acute Myocardial Infarction (AMI) went into atrial flutter with RVR post hip replacement 15 years ago and was anticoagulated and had bleeding. The number of patients with complications kept growing regardless of the patient's cardiac stability, risk score, or where he/she had surgery. These TJA patients had more complications than any of my cardiac patients undergoing noncardiac surgery.

During this time, there was an abrupt change in my practice model. The prior practice was based on echocardiography, stress echoes, single photon emission-computed tomography (SPECT) nuclear scans with exercise or chemical, cardiac catherization, stents, or bypass surgery. In 2004, my team gradually transitioned to 16 slice coronary computed tomographic angiography (CCTA)) , chemical Rb PET/CT scans, and cardiac magnetic resonance imaging with gadolinium as I discontinued diagnostic catheterization and stress testing, stress echo, and SPECT scanning. I hung up my catheters and quickly moved into a new era with encouragement and mentoring by Drs. Gerry Pohost, K. Lance Gould, Marcelo Di Carli, S. Dorbala, and Pim DeFeyter.

As we transitioned to 64 slice CCTA and HeartFlow, we gradually developed our own 5000 patient CT data base called Sherlock because we were contracted with IBM Watson to develop cardiac AI.

With this technology plus 4D echo with strain, our team became cardio-oncologists to diagnose and medically treat cancer patients who had potentially cardiotoxic cancer drug therapy or radiation therapy with a need to detect cardiac damage early and for prevention and treated. Because there was a need to grow these services internationally, our team became involved in the development of cardio-oncology internationally.

Physicians are well aware of the difficulty in making changes in medicine. The old adage is "tell me when you went to medical school and I'll tell you how you practice medicine." For example, it has been said that it took 17 years to get 60% of doctors to give a patient an aspirin who was having a heart attack (see Atul Gawande, "Checklist"). Why 17 years? The retirement/disability rate of practicing physicians is 6% per year. In 17 years at 6% per year, 102% of the physicians will turn over! That's a total replacement. But why only a 60% compliance with giving aspirin? We replaced the wrong doctors. We should have replaced the instructors whose retirement disability rate is only 4% per year whom it would take 25 years to replace.

But this time, we didn't have 25 years. So, the plan by our leadership was to put cardio-oncology into all the university medical schools by creating divisions, division heads, research grants, journals, and recruiting fellows. We should be able to establish significant change in practice in 8–9 years through the instructors, about one-third of the time taken for implementing only partial aspirin success. And we did! cardio-oncology is now in 50 universities in the United States and has developed about 15 international chapters.

Our team decided to apply the same logic to preoperative orthopedic patients by noninvasively using our advanced cardiac imaging technology to estimate their surgical risk anatomically rather than based on revised cardiac risk score (RCRI) historical information. We would do an echo, carotid ultrasound scan, abdominal aorta ultrasound, and CCTA to define the anatomy and thus better understand these patients' cardiac anatomy prior to TJA. Perhaps we could find untreated or unknown cardiac anatomical problems that may have an impact on risk. The application of this technology changed everything. We knew what the anatomical substrate was prior to surgery and could use this to guide new hypotheses concerning treatment decisions that might prevent cardiac perioperative problems as we are doing internationally in cardio-oncology.

As we started imaging these preoperative patients for TJA, there were quite a few surprises in this group with either known cardiovascular disease or patients with no cardiac histories all who were sent for preoperative cardiac clearance.

Patients were discovered to have left ventricular hypertrophy (LVH)) that was not known previously due to undiagnosed sleep apnea, inadequately controlled hypertension, or undiagnosed hypertension, all of which could be successfully treated preoperatively if we saw the patients at least a month before the surgical date. Patients with LVH and known hypertension on an medical regimen had their antihypertensive medications bumped up or new ones added. All LVH patients were monitored mostly by continuous rhythm monitoring for atrial fibrillation, and all newly discovered PAF/flutter patients were treated medically for prevention and anticoagulation depending on the CHADSVASC score. Antiarrhythmic medications were continued perioperatively including the day of surgery with sips of water.

After we predicted one of our patients was going to have a post-THA acute myocardial infarction based on his plaque morphology and composition, and rescued him with PTCA/stent in the LAD without myocardial damage, the largest private practice world class orthopedic group in Florida, the Florida Orthopaedic Institute, joined our efforts for TJA cardiac clearance using anatomical imaging information. This data was present at national and international orthopedic and cardiac meetings since these two specialties were in separate silos. Thus, cardio-orthopedics was launched. Our teams would follow our implementation of cardio-oncology as a bridge model for launching new technology and new concepts for quicker medical treatment assimilation across the health care enterprise! Centers for Medicare and Medicaid services (CMS)) bundling of cost of TJA provided an incentive for a cooperative effort to prevent readmission and resulted in alignment of cardiology and orthopedics.

This does not answer the question of why hip and knee replacement patients seem to have so many postoperative cardiac problems? Devereaux showed that of TJA patients over 65 y/o, 1/7 had elevated postop troponins (1). Is it the presence of chronic osteoarthritis as an inflammation that interacts with the cardiovascular system or is it the disability leading to less ambulation that promotes obesity, insulin resistance, hypertension, then LVH followed by PAF? If so, because most patients who have TJA are over 65 y/o, this older group should have more cardiovascular problems because of aging in association with progressive atherosclerosis.

THA is occurring at a younger age declining from 66 to just under 65 years of age and TKA age average declining from 68 to under 66 y/o. Is this group safer from cardiovascular risk? If these patients are getting TJA because of high performance athletics wear and tear of joints, a look at competitive and high-performance athletes may help us understand the younger patient risk.

For example, retired NFL players fit the profile of higher cardiac risk patients for TJA at a younger age. Not only do they have a greater need for TJA (11.4%) at a younger age, but they have the anatomical cardiac risk factors also at a younger age of LVH (1.5 × normal people with hypertension), which is associated with hypertension (45% of lineman), PAF(5.7 × greater chance), and sleep apnea (45% lineman and 35% non-lineman) making them not only prime targets for cardio-orthopedic evaluation but high profile individuals for being spokesmen for cardio-orthopedics.

It is my hope that this book will draw you into this circle of medical changers and care improvers embracing new technology, crossing silos and developing cognitive cardiology, as well as orthopedics as adeptly as we can currently add new apps to our patients' smart phones to improve their lives by accessing actionable data with greater ease.

Clinical Pearls:

Perioperative TJA CVAs are caused by PAF rather than cervical vascular disease. Patients with coronary artery disease can be sorted into those at low risk and high risk of cardiac events based on anatomy. Untreated or inadequately controlled hypertension are common.

Chapter Review Questions:

1. What is the number one postoperative non-orthopedic cause of complications in TJA patients over the age of 65? _____
2. What is the incidence of postoperative TJA over 65 y/o PAF?_____
3. CMS bundling of cost of TJA gave incentive to a cooperative effort to prevent readmission and resulted in alignment promoting silo bridging (T) or (F).

Total Joint Replacement, Contemporary Concepts

2

Thomas L. Bernasek, Meera Gill, Rajeev Herekar, and Steven T. Lyons

Abstract

In the 1960s, total hip replacement revolutionized management of elderly patients crippled with arthritis, with very good long-term results. Today, young patients present for hip-replacement surgery hoping to restore their quality of life, which typically includes physically demanding activities. Advances in bioengineering technology have driven development of hip prostheses. Both cemented and uncemented hips can provide durable fixation. Better materials and design have allowed use of large-bore bearings, which provide an increased range of motion with enhanced stability and very low wear. Minimally invasive surgery limits soft-tissue damage and facilitates accelerated discharge and rehabilitation. Short-term objectives must not compromise long-term performance. Computer-assisted surgery will contribute to reproducible and accurate placement of implants. Universal economic constraints in healthcare services dictate that further developments in total hip replacement will be governed by their cost-effectiveness. Over one million hip and knee joint replacements are performed each year, making it the third most commonly performed surgery in the United States (Etkin and Springer Arthroplast Today. 3:67–69, 2017). Recent data has shown long-term survivorship for total hip and knee arthroplasty to be 70.2% and 90.1% at 20 years, respectively (Chang and Haddad, Bone Joint J. 102-B(4):401–402, 2020). The demand for hip and knee joint replacement is driven by increased life expectancy and the arthritic patient's desire for pain relief, improved function, and quality of life. Demand for revision total joint arthroplasty, performed to repair a failed replacement is rising. This chapter reviews patient demographics, implant design, surgical techniques, and enabling technologies for joint replacement.

T. L. Bernasek (✉) · M. Gill · R. Herekar · S. T. Lyons
Florida Orthopedic Institute Group, Tampa, FL, USA

E. E. Harrison, N. H. Ho (eds.), *Managing Cardiovascular Risk In Elective Total Joint Arthroplasty*, https://doi.org/10.1007/978-3-031-26415-3_2

Keywords

Total joint arthroplasty (TJA) · Total hip arthroplasty (THA) · Coronary computed tomography angiography (CCTA) · Cardio-orthopedics

2.1 Case Report

Due to the age and comorbidities of many total joint replacement patients intersecting with value-based outcomes medical care, a premium is placed on avoidance of complications for these surgical patients. The following patient is an example where application of cardio-orthopedic principles can avoid perioperative events which increase the cost and prolong hospital stays.

MM is an 83-year-old female admitted on May 10 with a left femoral neck fracture after a fall at her assisted living facility. The fracture necessitated surgical intervention with a total hip replacement. Immediate preoperative medical ensued revealing a long-standing history of substernal chest pain. The patient had a cardiac stress test 3/2021 which raised concern for a "fixed defect," Therefore, cardiology was consulted pre op and since she had no chest pain, a non-ischemic EKG, and normal functional capacity was considered acceptable risk for surgery. Any other cardiac testing was deferred.

Uneventful total hip replacement was performed on May 11. On May 12, physical therapy ensued-she had orthostatic hypotension which resolved with IV fluids. On May 13, an echocardiogram was completed per cardiology demonstrating moderato-to-severe tricuspid valve regurgitation and a new diagnosis of pulmonary hypertension. Diuretics were not started due to orthostatic hypotension.

On May 14, she was transferred to the hospital in-patient rehabilitation center due to difficulty lifting and moving her right lower extremity (operative side). Postoperative films showed no change in her hip implant, therapy continued.

On May 21, post therapy in the rehab center, she reported chest heaviness. An initial EKG had "no changes." A follow-up EKG later that evening had ST elevation and labs showed elevated troponin (0.396). An urgent cardiology evaluation included bedside echocardiography demonstrating a large anterior wall motion abnormality. She was sent to CCU and on May 22 at 01:14 am to the Cath lab.

On May 22, she received two Xience stents to the LAD and was transferred back to CCU. She had new onset heart failure with an ejection fraction (EF) of 30–40% (EF May 21 was 60–65%).

On May 24, orthostatic hypotension limited ambulation. Meds adjusted by Cardiology.

5/25 cards started low-dose lopressor which improved her MAP, she began to tolerate therapy.

5/26 tolerating therapy, cardiac stable, transferred back to hospital rehab later this day.

5/29 continues in rehab, with BP 80s and lightheadedness, IVF given. Cardiology reconsulted to follow in rehab, lopressor dose decreased, f/u echo ordered.

5/31 echo resulted with improved EF 45–50%, rec to start midodrine to allow therapy tolerance.

6/3 advancing with therapy, with periods of fatigue, still with periods of dizziness dyspnea with am BM,

6/4 midodrine dose increased, Detrol started for urinary incontinence.

6–7 endurance and confidence improving with therapy, less urinary incontinence, family has arranged ATC care initially when returns to ALF, therapy will be provided by VNA. Plans are for discharge tomorrow on 6/8.

6–8 plans for discharge after 36 days of admission. Marked debilitation requiring ongoing and extensive physical therapy and home health services.

The above case report actually happened and represents a circumstance where an accurate diagnosis and preemptive cardiac treatment could obviate a cardiac event. For this patient, a hip joint replacement which typically requires 2–3 days admission resulted in a 26 day admission and extreme physical debilitation for the patient. The text which follows will discuss joint replacement and cardio-orthopedics. Cardio-orthopedics' goal is to facilitate early and accurate cardiac diagnosis in the vulnerable orthopedic patients in order to minimize cardiac-related complications and debilitation while facilitating a patient's rapid return to activity.

A. Introduction to total hip and total knee replacement
   (a) Asymptotical increase in the number of procedures for hip and knee replacement
   (b) Scope of the disease process, incidence, the percent of doctor office visits related to musculoskeletal disease, economic burden to society, the number of orthopedic procedures performed overall, the ranking of inpatient total hip and knee surgeries
   (c) Economics of total knee replacement and total hip replacement. Efforts to decrease costs including bundling, migration to outpatient surgery, improved efficiency for operative, and postoperative patient care

More than a million Americans have joint replacement surgery every year. This includes about 720,000 knee replacements and 330,000 hip replacements. Doctors also do this surgery on other joints like the shoulder and ankle. During this operation, the surgeon removes the damaged joint and replaces it with a new, artificial one. The surgeon may replace the entire joint or just part of it. People with joint damage, typically due to some form of arthritis, often have this operation. On average, joint replacement surgery ranges from $16,500–$33,000. Also known as joint arthroplasty, these highly effective treatments provide pain relief and functional improvement for patients with end-stage arthritis and are considered among the most successful surgeries in medicine. Recent data has shown long-term survivorship for total hip and knee arthroplasty to be 70.2% and 90.1% at 20 years, respectively [1]. The demand for hip and knee joint replacement is driven by increased life expectancy and the arthritic patient's desire for pain relief, improved function, and quality of life. Primary total hip arthroplasty is projected to grow by 174% and primary total knee arthroplasty by 673% by the year. Concurrently, demand for revision total joint arthroplasty, performed to repair a failed replacement is rising. Revision total hip arthroplasty is projected to grow by 137% and revision total knee arthroplasty by 601% by the year 2030 [2]. This chapter reviews patient demographics, implant design, surgical techniques, and enabling technologies for joint replacement. Later chapters will discuss patient selection and evaluation as medical comorbidity can increase the likelihood of complications which can result in patient death, disability, or implant failure, requiring revision.

Musculoskeletal disorders can be very painful and debilitating to quality of life. Affecting one in two people over age 18 years, and three in four people over age 65, musculoskeletal issues are one of the top reasons for a primary care or emergency department visit [3]. The knee is the most commonly affected joint followed by the hand and hip. The cost to treat the pain and disability from these conditions is rising rapidly. The average annual cost per person to treat musculoskeletal disorders is $7800. Annual US cost for treatment and lost wages has nearly doubled in less than two decades to $874 billion, or 5.7% of GDP [3].

Total hip and knee arthroplasty are among the most common orthopedic procedures performed. Osteoarthritis (OA), the most common type of arthritis, affects millions of people worldwide and is the most common indication for hip and knee arthroplasty. Other indications include hip fracture, rheumatoid arthritis, avascular necrosis, developmental dysplasia, Legg-Perthes disease and numerous others. OA is defined by an age-related "wear and tear" of the articular cartilage found in joints. Articular cartilage normally lines the ends of bones and provides a smooth surface for joint motion. Over time, this cartilage can break down and lead to changes in the exposed bone, tendon and ligament deterioration, and inflammation of the synovium, both at the surface and within the lining of the joints. This causes joint pain and stiffness and can result in disability. The knee is the most affected joint followed by the hand and hip. OA of the knee and hip can lead to severe pain and impairment of activities of daily life such as walking and using the bathroom. Unfortunately, it is a degenerative condition, and damage done to articular cartilage is irreversible. Therefore, the primary goals of managing a patient with severe osteoarthritis are pain relief, slowing disease progression disease, and improving function and quality of life. Nonsurgical methods of managing hip and knee osteoarthritis primarily address pain relief and disease progression. These methods include physical therapy, weight loss, and pain relief by use of oral medications, topical creams, or joint injections. If conservative methods fail, hip and knee arthroplasty are highly effective surgical methods for relieving pain and improving functional status [4].

Success for total hip and knee arthroplasty is high with respect to patient outcome and satisfaction [4]. A big factor in determining the success of these procedures, along with potential need for revision, is patient comorbidities. Common comorbidities seen in this patient population include hypertension, diabetes, obesity, depression, chronic pulmonary disease, hypothyroidism, and kidney disease, among others. Pre-existing cardiovascular disease, the leading cause of death in the United States, is associated with numerous adverse events after total joint replacement (TJR), including myocardial infarction (MI), congestive heart failure (CHF), symptomatic hypotension, pulmonary embolism (PE), and other cardiovascular complications [5]. Obesity, hypertension, and diabetes also demonstrate a particularly large effect on outcomes among patients requiring total hip, knee, or shoulder arthroplasty surgery, carrying a significant increase in postoperative complication rates and non-homebound disposition [6]. Obesity alone, affecting 42.4% of Americans (CDC 2018), is associated with significantly higher 30-day rates of wound complications, deep infection, reoperation rates, and total complications among total hip arthroplasty patients [7]. Patients with pulmonary hypertension suffer significantly more adverse events, including non-lethal cardiac dysrhythmias, morbidity rate, and longer hospital stays [8]. Patients with diabetes, including those with type II diabetes, those with diabetes for less than 5 years prior to surgery, those with complications due to diabetes, and those with cardiovascular comorbidities prior to surgery, have an increased risk of revision arthroplasty due to deep infection [9].

Total Hip Replacement

(a) The procedure and the implant alternatives
  (i) Discuss surgical approaches
    1. Direct anterior, anterior lateral, direct lateral, and posterior approach: define incidents of each and the potential positives of each approach include less common concepts including super cap approach
  (ii) Discuss implant design
    1. Traditional total hip replacement
    2. Resurfacing total hip replacement
    3. Advancements in design including highly cross-linked polyethylene, ceramics, bone in growth implant design versus cemented
  (iii) Discuss outcomes
    1. Focus on long-term outcomes
    2. Registry data might be useful

Dubbed "The Operation of the Century," total hip arthroplasty (THA) is one of the most effective and successful surgeries in medicine [4]. It has revolutionized the way an arthritic hip is treated and has helped millions of patients. As one of the largest joints in the body, the hip is a ball-and-socket joint where the head of the femur bone is a ball and the socket is formed by the acetabulum of the pelvis bone.

Several variations of hip arthroplasty exist. THA is a surgical procedure in which both the acetabulum and femoral head are replaced with prosthetic implants. The main indication for THA is severe, end-stage osteoarthritis, where the articular cartilage of the hip is worn away. THA can provide long-term pain relief, improvement in function and quality of life for patients suffering from osteoarthritis. Other indications for THA include avascular necrosis, trauma, tumors, and congenital hip disorders (Fig. 2.1).

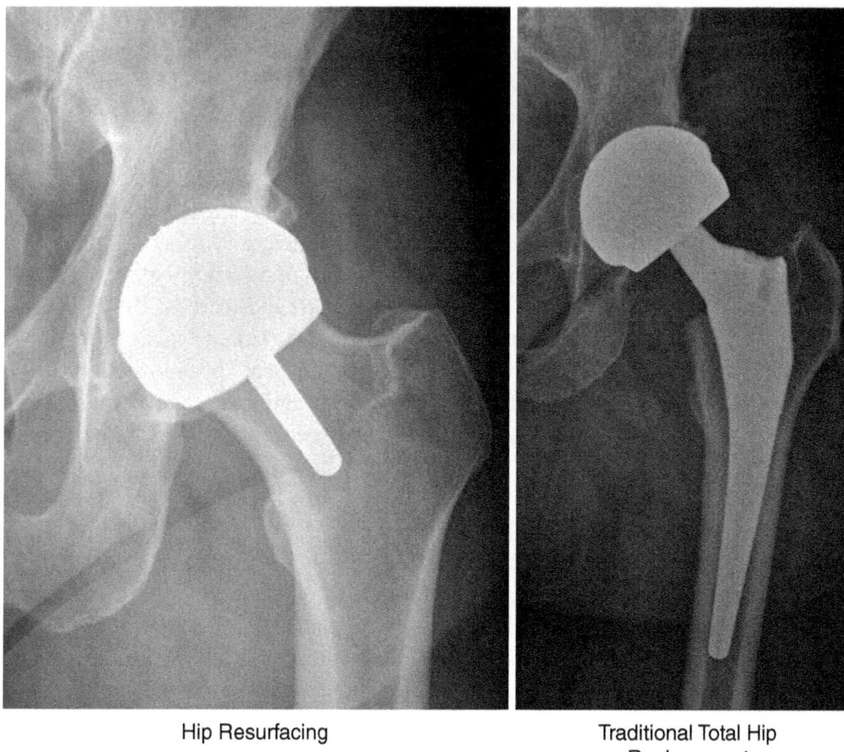

Fig. 2.1 On the left, the X-ray demonstrates hip resurfacing—note the large femoral head with a metal cap and a small stem within the intact femoral neck. On the right is a traditional THA implant with a smaller femoral head in contact with a polyethylene insert within the acetabular component seated on a monoblock stem

Resurfacing THA is a variation where the femoral head is resurfaced by capping the end of the bone and the acetabulum is resurfaced with a metal shell. Although this procedure preserves femoral bone, more acetabular bone removal is required. This is a metal-on-metal articulation which introduces the possibility of a metal-on-metal sensitivity reaction.

Hemiarthroplasty (monopolar or bipolar design) is performed to treat hip femoral neck fractures by replacing the femoral head only. It is typically indicated in low activity or high dislocation risk patients. This approach has the advantage of a more rapid surgery which is more stable to dislocation due to the use of a larger femoral head (increased head to neck ratio) and articulation with the native acetabulum. In order to dislocate, the femoral head must displace by half its diameter or more. One drawback is the potential for persistent pain due to acetabular cartilage wear and arthritis progression.

2.2 Surgical Approach

THA can be performed using a variety of surgical approaches to the hip joint. The most commonly used approaches include direct anterior, anterolateral, direct lateral, and posterior. Each approach has its advantages and disadvantages, and selection depends on multiple factors such as patient BMI, desired implant type, and surgeon experience. Any surgical approach can achieve an excellent THR result. The most important factor is surgeon experience. Due to direct-to-consumer marketing, the author has noted an increase in patient requests for the "anterior hip" approach because it does not violate any muscles. It is important that a patient trust the surgeon's choice of surgical approach as it is the one that he or she is most comfortable with. The imperative is proper implant placement. Some surgical approaches are referred to as "minimally invasive" procedures, which should be considered a marketing misnomer. Substantial implants are inserted to perform a hip replacement—this is far from minimally invasive. The focus of all hip replacement procedures is tissue preservation.

A direct anterior (DA) approach to the hip was described by Dr. Marius Nygaard Smith-Petersen in 1917 and is therefore sometimes known as the Smith-Petersen approach. A THR approach uses the distal limb of this approach which is considered the Huerter interval as described in 1882 [10]. It is considered a muscle-sparing approach since it exploits an intermuscular interval [11]. This anterior-based incision utilizes both intermuscular and internervous planes. Superficially, this plane consists of the tensor fascia lata (TFL) muscle, which is innervated by the superior gluteal nerve, and the sartorius muscle which is innervated by the femoral nerve. The deeper plane consists of the gluteus medius muscle which is innervated by the superficial gluteal nerve, and the rectus femoris muscle which is innervated by the femoral nerve. The procedure is performed in the supine position, often utilizing a table with attachments which enhance exposure. Advantages of this approach include a smaller incision, avoidance of the abductor mechanism, decreased dislocation rate, decreased pain, and earlier functional recovery. Disadvantages include a higher rate of intraoperative fracture, increased difficulty in very muscular or obese patients, increased surgical site infections rates in obese patients, the need for specialized hip implants and lateral femoral cutaneous nerve injury.

The anterolateral or Watson-Jones approach was popularized by Sir Watson Jones in the 1930s and has many similarities to the direct anterior approach. The procedure can be performed with the patient in the supine or lateral position and does not require a specialized table. The intermuscular plane utilized is between the TFL and gluteus medius, both which are innervated by the superior gluteal nerve. Advantages to this approach include a lower dislocation rate when compared to the posterior approach and unlikely to injure the lateral femoral cutaneous nerve. Disadvantages include increased difficulty in very muscular patients.

The direct lateral approach is the second most common approach for a THA. It is often referred to as the "Hardinge" approach as it was first described by Dr.

Hardinge in 1982. This approach elevates a portion of the gluteus medius and the gluteus minimus from the proximal femur for exposure and capsulotomy. These structures are firmly repaired after hip prosthesis implantation. A significant benefit to this approach is a low rate of postoperative dislocation when compared to the other approaches. This is due to the preservation of the hip posterior capsule and short external rotator muscle attachments. This approach can also be easily extended should further exposure be needed. A potential superior gluteal nerve injury is a disadvantage of this approach, which can lead to abductor muscle weakness resulting in a limp.

The posterior approach is the most widely used surgical approach for THA. Called a "Southern" or "Moore" approach as it was popularized by Dr. A.T. Moore in 1957. The posterior approach splits the gluteus maximus muscle, exposing the posterior hip capsule and short external rotators which are dissected and detached. The posterior approach is popular because it does not disrupt the abductor mechanism and can easily be extended proximally and distally for more exposure. However, it has a historically higher rate of postoperative dislocation when compared to the other surgical approaches, and the sciatic nerve is more vulnerable to injury.

New techniques supporting novel hip implant designs have been released in the quest to improve patient outcome and function. For example, the recently introduced supercapsular approach utilizes the interval between the gluteus medius and piriformis muscles to access the hip capsule. This method attempts to preserve the external rotators and the capsule, hopefully reducing postoperative pain and accelerating postoperative function. Reported disadvantages to this approach include implant malpositioning from the limited femoral exposure. As with many newer techniques, this lacks long-term outcome studies.

Computer-assisted navigation and robotic surgery are more recent techniques being utilized to improve the accuracy of implant placement and to reduce surgical error in THA. Computer-assisted navigation surgery begins with a Computed Tomography (CT) or MRI scan of a patient's limb which is fed into a computer. Trackers are placed into the patient's pelvis and femur. Computer software provides the surgeon with accurate, real-time information to guide bone cuts and implant placement. Recent innovations can provide reliable surgical assistance using only intraoperative plain X-rays and a computer analysis of implant placement as a guide (e.g., JointPoint™).

Robotic surgery combines computer-assisted navigation with a robotic device that assists a surgeon to execute a planned bone resection and implant positioning. A surgeon is present to define, confirm, and guide bone cuts and implant placement. Most major implant manufacturers have or are developing a robotic system. These systems utilize a robotic arm for cutting or milling bone or a system for accurate placement of cutting jigs or implants. This technology can increase accuracy and decrease variability. Robotic technology in the field of joint arthroplasty is promising however current limitations of high cost and lack of long-term outcome data exist. The perceived benefits of improved and consistent accuracy will likely prevail and the technology will continue to expand.

2.3 Implant Design

Hip replacement design has improved steadily since the first reported ivory femoral head hip arthroplasty in 1802 by Dr. Themistocles Gluck. Low friction total hip arthroplasty using a metallic femoral stem with a small femoral head and a cemented polyethylene acetabular cup was introduced in the 1960s by Sir John Charnley and has shaped modern THA. While the early results of Charnley's designs were poor, the concepts he developed have influenced THA techniques and implants since.

Most modern THA designs are modular and assembled intraoperatively. These implant designs have four components: the acetabular cup, acetabular liner, femoral head, and femoral stem. Typical materials for the acetabular cup and femoral stem are titanium or cobalt-chromium alloys with a polyethylene or ceramic liner. Both the acetabular cup and femoral stem can be implanted with or without cement, with cementless fixation most common. Cementless implants have a porous or grit-blasted surface for patient bone attachment. This is known as biological fixation, and the implant is often referred to as a press-fit implant. Cementless fixation is widely successful but includes the risk of fracture during placement due to the tight fit required to achieve initial rigid fixation.

The second most common method for hip implant fixation is cementation. Cement provides good initial and long-term stability but requires additional surgical time for the cement to dry. Typically, it is used in patients with marked osteopenia, severe bone loss, or pathologic bone which does not provide adequate support for a cementless implant. During cement insertion and pressurization, circulating cement monomers can provoke cardiopulmonary collapse and death. This infrequent event is most common in those with underlying cardiac or pulmonary comorbidities and dehydration. Patient medical optimization prior to and during surgery is important for those undergoing cemented fixation.

Improved bearing surface technology has significantly increased hip implant longevity. The bearing surface consists of a femoral head articulating with the acetabular liner and can be made of either polyethylene, ceramic, or metal. Four commonly used combinations for the femoral head and acetabular bearing surface, respectively, are metal on polyethylene, metal on metal, ceramic on polyethylene, and ceramic on ceramic. Each combination has its advantages and disadvantages.

Metal on polyethylene has the longest track record of all the bearing surfaces available. It has shown good long-term results and is the least expensive choice. However, when compared to other material combinations, early polyethylene designs had very high wear and osteolysis rates. Implant wear has been dramatically reduced by the development of highly cross-linked polyethylene. This type of polyethylene is a highly wear-resistant material which has decreased osteolysis rates dramatically. For this reason, it is now the most commonly used acetabular bearing surface.

Metal on metal bearings were introduced to avoid the complications of polyethylene wear and osteolysis. While initial outcomes showed significantly reduced wear rates and increased hip stability, problems began to arise when some patients developed metal hypersensitivity reactions such as adverse local tissue reactions leading to pseudo tumors, and tissue destruction. The increased failure rates led to metal-on-metal bearings falling out of favor.

Ceramic is harder with better lubricity than metal and therefore has the best wear rate of all materials. It has been shown to perform well, having low revision rates and wear-related problems, especially when paired with highly cross-linked polyethylene. Over the last 8 years, there has been an increase in ceramic on polyethylene combinations while metal on polyethylene has declined. Ceramic on ceramic bearings, however, have been limited by their expensive cost and complications that include implant squeaking and very rarely, fracture.

Hip resurfacing arthroplasty (HRA) is an alternative method to conventional total hip arthroplasty. The surgical approach to the hip is similar to that used in THA; however, the entire femoral head and neck are not removed. Instead, the femoral head is resurfaced with a metal cap creating a metal-on-metal implant. Advantages of this procedure includes proximal femur bone preservation, a low dislocation rate, minimized stress shielding and in many cases can be easily revised using a primary femoral component. Potential disadvantages include femoral neck fracture, early implant failure, and metal sensitivity reactions. Factors including increased patient age, female sex, and poor bone stock have been shown to contribute to HRA failure. Therefore, this technique is indicated primarily for male patients less than 60 years of age with good bone stock.

2.4 Outcomes

THA is one of the most effective and successful surgical procedures available in medicine. Outcomes are generally excellent and highly reproducible. Per available registry data, most hip replacements have a lifespan of 15–20 years, and over 90% of patients report achieving a meaningful improvement after undergoing primary THA. Despite the success of THA, research continues to find new surgical approaches, techniques, and implant designs to improve implant longevity, patient outcome and to accelerate recovery.

B. Total knee replacement
   (a) The procedure and implant alternatives
      (i) Total knee replacement versus partial knee replacement, including patellofemoral
      (ii) Surgical approaches and techniques
         1. Medial peripatellar, lateral approach, subvastus approach
         2. Advanced instrumentation, robotics, sensor technology
         3. Implant design advancements including sizing, kinematics, implant fixation (cementless versus cemented), polyethylene improvements including cross-linking, conformity, and mobile bearing

(iii) Discuss outcomes
   1. Focus on long-term outcomes
   2. Registry data might be useful

There are numerous nonoperative methods for knee arthritis such as exercise, nonsteroidal anti-inflammatory drugs (NSAIDs), and injections. However, when these treatments are ineffective, a popular and widely successful surgical option is total knee replacement. There are multiple treatment options within this category depending on a patient's scope of disease including total knee replacement and unicompartmental or partial knee replacement.

The knee is a complex hinge joint with many ligaments, tendons, and muscles that create stability and support throughout knee motion and activity. Total knee replacement (TKR) must allow near-normal flexion, extension, and rotation while addressing the pain and arthritis of the patellofemoral and tibiofemoral joints. In addition, a TKR must tolerate the significant forces generated at the patellofemoral joint by the extensor mechanism and at the tibiofemoral joint which transmits body weight from the femur to tibia. The maximum contact force of the patellofemoral joint, for example, can be up to 7.8 times bodyweight in a deep squat [12, 13], while the maximum contact force of the tibiofemoral joint has been measured at 5.1 times bodyweight while running [14].

2.5 Surgical Approach

Total knee arthroplasty (TKA) is the most commonly performed joint arthroplasty surgery [15]. TKA is highly effective at restoring function and relieving pain for patients suffering from end-stage arthritis. There are four popular surgical approaches to a total or partial knee arthroplasty. These include the medial parapatellar, subvastus, midvastus, and lateral approaches, each named for the location of the arthrotomy or opening of the joint capsule. The medial parapatellar approach is the most used. Typically, a midline, anterior skin incision extends from the tibial tuberosity distally to above the patella proximally. Once subcutaneous tissue and fascia have been dissected, an arthrotomy is performed. Dislocation and eversion of the patella permits surgical preparation and exposure for the rest of the knee joint.

Implant alignment and ligament balancing are critical to TKR function and outcome. Sophisticated instrumentation guides bone cuts for optimal component placement. Burgeoning computer technology employing robotic-assisted devices for implant alignment, ligament balancing, and bone cuts are now coming onto the TKR scene. Each of the major implant manufacturers now offers robots including Mako™ (Stryker), Velys™ (Depuy/J&J), ROSA™ (Zimmer/Biomet), Navio™ (Smith & Nephew), and OMNI™ (Corin). These devices improve the accuracy of component alignment. To date, improved alignment resulting in improved function and outcomes has not justified the increased cost and operative time associated with robotic surgery. Surgeon acceptance of this new technology continues to increase as the technology improves.

2.6 Implant Design

Modern TKA implants resurface the bones of the knee via femoral, tibial, and patellar components that are placed after precise bone removal—typically a 9 mm segment. The implant itself can be categorized into three main designs which are implemented depending on patient factors and surgeon preference. These designs, in order of increasing level of constraint, or stabilization, are cruciate-retaining, posterior-stabilized, and constrained.

Cruciate retaining (CR) TKA designs are the least constrained and are utilized in patients with an intact posterior cruciate ligament (PCL). The primary function of the PCL is to prevent excessive posterior tibial translation relative to femur. PCL retention preserves distal femoral bone stock and knee kinematics in a properly designed TKR. CR TKA surgical technique must avoid a PCL that is too tight or too loose to optimize function.

Posterior-stabilized (PS) or semi-constrained TKR requires PCL removal and replaces its function with a cam and post. The femoral component has a housing with a cam designed to engage a post on the tibial polyethylene bearing. This design is slightly more constrained than a CR TKA. An advantage to a PS TKA is that the knee is easier to balance with an absent PCL. Disadvantages include cam and post complications and increased femoral bone resection.

Constrained TKA designs are indicated for knee instability due to ligament deficiency. Moderate to massive bone loss is often present and must be accommodated by the knee design. Implants utilize a large tibial post and deep femoral box, or for severe instability, a hinged design. Both non-hinged and hinged constrained designs have the disadvantage of possible early aseptic loosening due to the increased constraint which increases stress on the implant fixation. Significant femoral bone resection is often required for these implants. Fortunately, constrained designs are most commonly seen in complex or revision TKA.

A significant factor in the success and longevity of TKR is modern polyethylene. To prevent oxidation which degrades polyethylene strength, highly cross-linked polyethylene with antioxidants has been developed. This cross-linked, antioxidant-laden poly has dramatically improved wear with an expected service life measured in decades (Bryan et al.). Some implant designs utilize mobile-bearing polyethylene which further decreases wear. Such designs are indicated for younger, active patients.

Unicompartmental or partial knee replacement (UKA) is an option for osteoarthritis affecting only one compartment of the knee. UKR makes up about 5% of all knee replacements. In properly selected patients, UKA provides satisfactory outcomes with a quicker recovery and a more natural feeling knee due to retention of normal ligaments and cartilage. The medial compartment is most commonly affected and replaced. Early results for UKA showed high failure rates due to aseptic loosening and fractures. However, newer modifications, techniques, and interest in minimally invasive options have led to much better outcomes. UKA implants demonstrate good survivorship rates with 95% and 90% at 10 and 20 years, respectively (Foran et al.).

Patients who suffer from isolated patellofemoral joint arthritis have the option of a kneecap replacement. Replacing only the kneecap allows for preservation of the tibiofemoral joint, leading to faster recovery and satisfactory outcomes.

TKR and UKR fixation can be cemented or uncemented. The cemented fixation method is used by the majority of surgeons as it provides excellent outcomes. This method uses polymethylmethacrylate to adhere the implant to bone. Cement works well for patients who have poor bone quality and allows for immediate fixation, so patients can bear weight right after surgery. Although aseptic loosening can occur over time, the incidence is relatively low and will likely decrease further with modern implants.

Uncemented TKR uses implants with a porous surface that allows bone ingrowth and attachment directly to the implant. This biological fixation requires the implant to have properties and pore size that resembles normal trabecular bone. Although complete healing of the bone attachment can take as long as 2 years, immediate weight bearing and knee function is possible.

2.7 Outcomes

C. Complications following total hip and total knee arthroplasty
   (a) Discuss the full gamut of possible complications, lead into the medical complications, and in particular, cardiac, which will be the focus of subsequent chapters.

Total hip and knee arthroplasty are widely considered as safe and effective procedures. However, despite clinical success of these procedures, medical complications following total hip and knee arthroplasty can occur in any patient and range from minor to life-threatening events. Risk for these complications is especially high in older patients with comorbidities. Since TJR is an elective procedure, patient selection and medical optimization prior to surgery is imperative.

Surgical complications that can occur following THA and TKA include bone fractures, dislocation or subluxation, surgical site bleeding, and infection.

Pulmonary complications after THA and TKA. While obesity is not a contraindication to total joint arthroplasty, patients in this demographic who undergo THA have drastically increased periprosthetic complications such as a two-fold increase in hip dislocation, increased wound dehiscence, periprosthetic joint infection, acute renal failure, revision arthroplasty, and death (Meller et al.). Glycemic control among diabetics is also evaluated prior to total joint replacement as an HbA1C level greater than 7.7% has been strongly associated with periprosthetic joint infection and other complications (Tarabichi et al). Additionally, preoperative nutrition status is an important factor to consider among prospective total joint patients, with albumin values less than 3.0 being associated with significantly increased postoperative complications and poor wound healing (Nelson et al.) [17–39].

Cardiovascular complications following THA and TKA are a major cause of morbidity and mortality, representing 20% of all major postoperative complications. These complications include venous thromboembolic events such as deep vein thrombosis (DVT), pulmonary embolism (PE), myocardial infarction, cerebrovascular accidents, and acute renal failure. A history of cardiac disease and older age have been identified as two significant risk factors for developing cardiac complications postoperatively. Additional risk factors include renal failure, anemia, smoking history, bilateral arthroplasty, cerebrovascular disease, and ASA class. While these risk factors have been shown to lead to cardiac complications, there is inconsistency regarding which of these factors are important predictors of complications. In addition, no preoperative risk stratification tool exists to determine which risk factors that deem cardiac optimization necessary prior to THA or TKA. The subsequent chapters of this textbook aim to address these inconsistencies and help cardiologists and orthopedic surgeons understand cardiovascular perioperative risk in patients undergoing THA and TKA.

References

1. Chang JS, Haddad FS. Long-term survivorship of hip and knee arthroplasty. Bone Joint J. 2020;102-B(4):401–2. https://doi.org/10.1302/0301-620x.102b4.bjj-2020-0183.
2. Kurtz S, Ong K, Lau E, Mowat F, Halpern M. Projections of primary and revision hip and knee arthroplasty in the United States from 2005 to 2030. J Bone Joint Surg Am. 2007;89(4):780–5. https://doi.org/10.2106/JBJS.F.00222.
3. United States Bone and Joint Initiative. The burden of musculoskeletal diseases in the United States (BMUS). 4th ed. Rosemont, IL: United States Bone and Joint Initiative; 2020. http://www.boneandjointburden.org
4. Learmonth ID, Young C, Rorabeck C. The operation of the century: total hip replacement. Lancet. 2007;370(9597):1508–19. https://doi.org/10.1016/s0140-6736(07)60457-7.
5. Basilico FC, Sweeney G, Losina E, Gaydos J, Skoniecki D, Wright EA, Katz JN. Risk factors for cardiovascular complications following total joint replacement surgery. Arthritis Rheum. 2008;58(7):1915–20. https://doi.org/10.1002/art.2360739.
6. Jain NB, Guller U, Pietrobon R, Bond TK, Higgins LD. Comorbidities increase complication rates in patients having arthroplasty. Clin Orthop Relat Res. 2005;435:232–8. https://doi.org/10.1097/01.blo.0000156479.97488.a2.
7. DeMik DE. Complications and obesity in arthroplasty—a hip is not a Knee. J Arthroplast. 2018;33(10):3281–7. https://doi.org/10.1016/j.arth.2018.02.073. Epub 2018 Feb 26. https://pubmed.ncbi.nlm.nih.gov/29631859/
8. Kim D, Jules-Elysee K, Turteltaub L, Urban MK, YaDeau JT, Reid S, Lyman S, Ma Y. Clinical outcomes in patients with pulmonary hypertension undergoing total hip arthroplasty. HSS J. 2014;10(2):131–5. https://doi.org/10.1007/s11420-014-9391-y.
9. Pedersen AB, Mehnert F, Johnsen SP, Sørensen HT. Risk of revision of a total hip replacement in patients with diabetes mellitus. J Bone Surg Brit. 2010;92–B(7):929–34. https://doi.org/10.1302/0301-620x.92b7.24461.
10. Petis S, Howard JL, Lanting BL, Vasarhelyi EM. Surgical approach in primary total hip arthroplasty: anatomy, technique and clinical outcomes. Can J Surg. 2015;58(2):128–39. https://doi.org/10.1503/cjs.007214.
11. Moskal JT. Anterior muscle sparing approach for total hip arthroplasty. World J Orthop. 2013;4(1):12. https://doi.org/10.5312/wjo.v4.i1.12.

12. Flynn TW, Soutas-Little RW. Patellofemoral joint compressive forces in forward and backward running. J Orthop Sports Phys Ther. 1995;21(5):277–82. https://doi.org/10.2519/jospt.1995.21.5.277.
13. Huberti HH, Hayes WC. Patellofemoral contact pressures. The influence of q-angle and Tendofemoral contact. J Bone Surg. 1984;66(5):715–24. https://doi.org/10.2106/00004623-198466050-00010.
14. Saxby DJ, Modenese L, Bryant AL, Gerus P, Killen B, Fortin K, Wrigley TV, Bennell KL, Cicuttini FM, Lloyd DG. Tibiofemoral contact forces during walking, running and sidestepping. Gait Posture. 2016;49:78–85. https://doi.org/10.1016/j.gaitpost.2016.06.014.
15. American Joint Replacement Registry (AJRR). 2020 Annual Report. Rosemont, IL: American Academy of Orthopaedic Surgeons (AAOS); 2020.
16. Etkin CD, Springer BD. The American joint replacement registry—the first 5 years. Arthroplast Today. 2017;3(2):67–9. 2017. https://doi.org/10.1016/j.artd.2017.02.002.
17. Sheth D, Cafri G, Inacio MC, Paxton EW, Namba RS. Anterior and anterolateral approaches for THA are associated with lower dislocation risk without higher revision risk. Clin Orthop Relat Res. 2015;473(11):3401–8. https://doi.org/10.1007/s11999-015-4230-0.
18. Blankstein M, Lentine B, Nelms NJ. The use of cement in hip arthroplasty: a contemporary perspective. J Am Acad Orthop Surg. 2020;28(14):e586–94. https://doi.org/10.5435/JAAOS-D-19-00604.
19. Donaldson AJ, et al. Bone cement implantation syndrome. Br J Anaesth. 2009;102(1):12–22.
20. Lee JM. The current concepts of Total hip arthroplasty. Hip Pelvis. 2016;28(4):191–200. https://doi.org/10.5371/hp.2016.28.4.191.
21. Galia CR, Diesel CV, Guimarães MR, Ribeiro TA. Total hip arthroplasty: a still evolving technique. Rev Bras Ortop. 2017;52(5):521–7. https://doi.org/10.1016/j.rboe.2016.09.011.
22. Hu CY, Yoon TR. Recent updates for biomaterials used in total hip arthroplasty. Biomater Res. 2018;22:33. https://doi.org/10.1186/s40824-018-0144-8.
23. Mont MA, Ragland PS, Etienne G, Seyler TM, Schmalzried TP. Hip resurfacing arthroplasty. J Am Acad Orthop Surg. 2006;14(8):454–63.
24. Sershon R, Balkissoon R, Valle CJ. Current indications for hip resurfacing arthroplasty in 2016. Curr Rev Musculoskelet Med. 2016;9(1):84–92. https://doi.org/10.1007/s12178-016-9324-0.
25. Kayani B, Konan S, Ayuob A, Ayyad S, Haddad FS. The current role of robotics in total hip arthroplasty. EFORT Open Rev. 2019;4(11):618–25. https://doi.org/10.1302/2058-5241.4.180088.
26. Sugano N. Computer-assisted orthopaedic surgery and robotic surgery in total hip arthroplasty. Clin Orthop Surg. 2013;5(1):1–9. https://doi.org/10.4055/cios.2013.5.1.1. Epub 2013 Feb 20. PMID: 23467021; PMCID: PMC3582865
27. Wilhelm SK, Henrichsen JL, Siljander M, Moore D, Karadsheh M. Polyethylene in total knee arthroplasty: where are we now? J Orthop Surg. 2018;26:2309499018808356. https://doi.org/10.1177/2309499018808356.
28. Peters CL, Mulkey P, Erickson J, Anderson MB, Pelt CE. Comparison of total knee arthroplasty with highly congruent anterior-stabilized bearings versus a cruciate-retaining design. Clin Orthop Relat Res. 2014;472(1):175–80. https://doi.org/10.1007/s11999-013-3068-6.
29. Dall'Oca C, Ricci M, Vecchini E, et al. Evolution of TKA design. Acta Biomed. 2017;88(2S):17–31. https://doi.org/10.23750/abm.v88i2-S.6508.
30. Campi S, Tibrewal S, Cuthbert R, Tibrewal SB. Unicompartmental knee replacement—current perspectives. J Clin Orthop Trauma. 2018;9(1):17–23. https://doi.org/10.1016/j.jcot.2017.11.013.
31. Belmont PJ, Goodman GP, Kusnezov NA, Magee C, Bader JO, Waterman BR, et al. Postoperative myocardial infarction and cardiac arrest following primary total knee and hip arthroplasty: rates, risk factors, and time of occurrence. J Bone Joint Surg (Am Vol). 2014;96(24):2025–31. https://doi.org/10.2106/JBJS.N.00153.
32. Elsiwy Y, Jovanovic I, Doma K, Hazratwala K, Letson H. Risk factors associated with cardiac complication after total joint arthroplasty of the hip and knee: a systematic review. J Orthop Surg Res. 2019;14(1):15. https://doi.org/10.1186/s13018-018-1058-9.

33. Elsiwy Y, Symonds T, Doma K, Hazratwala K, Wilkinson M, Letson H. Pre-operative clinical predictors for cardiology referral prior to total joint arthroplasty: the 'asymptomatic' patient. J Orthop Surg Res. 2020;15(1):513. https://doi.org/10.1186/s13018-020-02042-5.
34. Mary Elizabeth Dallas The 10 Most Common Surgeries in the U.S. Healthgrades Website. 2019. https://www.healthgrades.com/explore/the-10-most-common-surgeries-in-the-us. Accessed 28 Dec 2020
35. Nedopil AJ, Singh AK, Howell SM, Hull ML. Does calipered kinematically aligned Tka restore native left to RIGHT symmetry of the lower limb and improve function? J Arthroplast. 2018;33(2):398–406. https://doi.org/10.1016/j.arth.2017.09.039.
36. American Joint Replacement Registry. Annual Report 2019. (n.d.). https://www.aaos.org/globalassets/registries/2020-aaos-ajrr-annual-report-preview_final.pdf.
37. Crosby Kyle D. Titanium-6Aluminum-4Vanadium for functionally graded orthopedic implant applications (2013). Doctoral Dissertations 218. https://opencommons.uconn.edu/dissertations/218
38. AO Surgery Reference. Arthroplasty (2010). https://surgeryreference.aofoundation.org/orthopedic-trauma/adult-trauma/proximal-femur/femoral-neck-fracture-transcervical-or-basicervical/arthroplasty?searchurl=%2fSearchResults#total-hip-replacement
39. Nguyen D. Simulation and experimental study on polishing of SPHERICAL steel by non-Newtonian fluids. Int J Adv Manuf Technol. 2020;107(1–2):763–73. https://doi.org/10.1007/s00170-020-05055-w.

3 Impact of CMS Mandatory and Volunteer Bundle Total Joint Arthroplasty Care and How This Has Created New Models for Inpatient Surgery

Kenneth Gustke and Penny Boness

Abstract

Bundled risk plans for medical care is becoming more prevalent as Medicare and private insurance plans note significant savings. These programs require management of all aspects of an episode of care by the physician group or hospital that owns the bundle. Our experience in managing the Bundled Payments for Care Improvement Program (BPCI) Model 2 and how it has produced significant cost savings and improved patient care are discussed.

Keywords

Bundled Payments for Care Improvement Program (BPCI) · Comprehensive Care for Joint Replacement Model bundle (CJR) · Center for Medicare and Medicaid Services, Center for Medicare and Medicaid Innovation (CMS)

K. Gustke (✉)
Adult Reconstruction and Arthritis Surgery of the Hip and Knee, Florida Orthopaedic Institute, Temple Terrace, FL, USA

Clinical Professor of Orthopedic Surgery, Department of Orthopedic Surgery, University of South Florida College of Medicine, Tampa, FL, USA
e-mail: KGustke@floridaortho.com

P. Boness
Florida Orthopaedic Institute, Temple Terrace, FL, USA
e-mail: pboness@floridaortho.com

E. E. Harrison, N. H. Ho (eds.), *Managing Cardiovascular Risk In Elective Total Joint Arthroplasty*, https://doi.org/10.1007/978-3-031-26415-3_3

3.1 Case

A 78-year-old female had severe osteoarthritis of her right hip with significant dysfunction. She had exhausted non-operative treatment and was recommended a total hip replacement. She would be part of a Medicare bundled payment risk program. She was 4′11″ tall, weighed 184 lbs., with a BMI of 37.2. She had severe osteoarthritis of her right hip. Her admitted medical problems were hypothyroidism, hypertension, and a previous lower extremity deep venous thrombosis. Medications included paroxetine, ranitidine, levothyroxine, zolpidem, metoprolol, ibuprofen, and oxycodone. She denied any cardiac disease, but a pre-operative cardiac workup was requested. Tests included an electrocardiogram, echocardiogram, carotid ultrasound, coronary computed tomography angiography, and a 3-day cardiac rhythm monitor. She was found to have uncontrolled hypertension, 60% left ventricular hypertrophy, an ejection fraction of 64%, mild disease in left anterior descending coronary artery, and intermittent atrial fibrillation. Because atrial fibrillation frequently leads to a readmission, it was aggressively treated. She was placed on nebivolol, apixaban, dronedarone, and ranolazine. She was cleared to proceed with total hip replacement surgery. A total hip replacement surgery was performed with no complications.

3.2 Background

Classically, physicians are paid for patient care by a fee-for-service model. Because payment for services are given separately to hospitals, physicians, and rehabilitation providers, there is minimal accountability from one provider to the others to coordinate care, optimize outcome, and hold down costs. In a fee-for-service model, the physician orders the treatment, but has no incentive to minimize the use of expensive or perhaps unnecessary treatment. Because the physician is not required to control the quality of care given by other providers, they are not able to guarantee a quality result. Bundled Payments for Care Improvement Program (BPCI) Model 2 was developed in 2013 by the US Center for Medicare and Medicaid Innovation (CMS) as a service delivery model for an acute and post-acute care episode whereby an awarded organization accepts financial liability and performance accountability. The purpose was to promote coordinated care via risk sharing to reduce costs while maintaining quality.

In a bundled service model, one entity takes charge of a finite episode of care. The BPCI Model 2 program was available to physician groups or hospitals to manage an episode of care for a specific period of time. Reducing costs for hip and knee replacement surgery is especially desirable to Medicare since they represent the highest expense of any inpatient procedure [1]. For the orthopedic hip and knee arthroplasty program, all patients who underwent elective or unplanned standard Medicare total hip and knee replacement (DRG 470) and replacements for hip fracture (DRG 469) surgeries had to be enrolled. The manager of the episode of care would be responsible to coordinate the inpatient and post-discharge care for 90 days.

The total 90-day expenditures were reconciled against the provider's historic average cost. Part of any savings under the historic target price would provide for a monetary bonus to the managing group. If costs were higher, a portion would be deducted from the surgical fee payment to the orthopedic surgeon. A convener was required to act as a liaison between the providers and CMS.

Opportunities for cost savings could occur by reducing unnecessary initial hospital costs, readmissions, inpatient rehabilitation stays, skilled nursing stays, home health visits, and outpatient physical therapy visits, all without decreasing outcomes. The quality metrics that had to be met include a lower 30-day readmission rate. Readmission after total hips and knee arthroplasty are common and especially costly to managers of a risk adjusted bundled payment program [2]. A pre-operative assessment and education was required on every patient. The patient had to be informed and engaged with the program and care plan.

The risk that bundled payment programs can create to the US health care system is that the incentive to reduce care to save costs and provide the provider with a bonus could lessen the quality of care. Hospital stays could be unsafely shortened or typical post-discharge care could be denied. The patient may feel that they have received less care than they otherwise would have been entitled to under a classic fee-for-service model. This can be mitigated by agreeing on expectations preoperatively and delivering an acceptable patient satisfaction level. Another risk is that this program would save overall cost to Medicare and increase bonuses to the provider by simply denying access to care to high-risk patients. However, providers would ideally just delay care in order to optimize the health of the patient by eliminating modifiable risk factors or improving uncorrectable risk factors, and ultimately still provide the care for the high-risk patient.

Reported studies with bundled programs have demonstrated a significant cost savings to Medicare without a significant decrease in quality of care and only slight decrease in patient satisfaction [3–5]. Savings have occurred by reducing hospital length of stay, more discharges to home, and lower readmissions [6–8]. Patients of lower socioeconomic status have been shown to have a higher risk of needing greater post-hospital rehabilitation and have higher readmission rates [9].

3.3 Requirements for Successful Participation in a Risk Bundle Program

Every stage of the 90-day care event has to be monitored. Physicians have to work with the hospitals to develop standardized care plans to hopefully reduce complications, length of stay, and overall costs. A preferred network of skilled nursing facilities, home health care agencies, and outpatient physical therapy facilities needs to be developed. These relationships allowed for consistent care plans, goals, and expectations to be established with these medical providers to better manage patient care, prohibit unnecessary visits, and recommend discharge when appropriate.

Case managers were hired by the practice specifically to coordinate the care of patients in this program. They needed to have direct contact with patients pre-operatively to develop a contract with expectations and a discharge plan. The patients need to be assured that they would have an excellent outcome without the need to utilize maximum Medicare allowed rehabilitation days in most cases. Waiver assistance at the practices expense such as house sitters, pet sitters, and transportation could also be arranged to allow shorter inpatient and skilled nursing stays. The case manager would become the primary point of contact for the patients so they would be called first with questions and concerns. They would then be directed to appropriate care and hopefully avoid emergency room visits. The patients appreciated this easy access. The case managers would then follow the patient's progress while in rehabilitation facilities, receiving home health, and outpatient physical therapy. They were also in contact with the medical providers to make sure appropriate progress is occurring without unnecessary stays and visits. Everyone touching the patient needs to be on board with the program.

The patients needed to be medically optimized preoperatively via appropriate screening and other medical consultations. The dilemma is that the orthopedic surgeon is placed in a position to minimize postoperative medical complications in a higher risk population in fields outside their discipline. We previously would ask the patient's primary care physician to preoperatively medically clear the patient for surgery. They could decide whether a cardiology evaluation was necessary. Cardiac complications are one of highest cause of serious complications after total hip and knee replacement. Osteoarthritic patients commonly have unrecognized cardiac symptoms masked by their inactivity. We noted that an EKG was the usual screening tool by primary care physician and even many cardiologists to clear the patient for surgery. Analysis of 337 of our Medicare patients undergoing primary hip and knee replacement surgery prior to our involvement in BPCI showed only 4 (1.2%) patients were readmitted for a cardiac complication. However, the average readmission hospital stay was 3.33 days with a total cost for readmission for these patients of $42,321. As a result of this data, we determined that the patient's orthopedic surgeon was required to take more active role in directing preoperative medical optimization in risk bundled programs. We required a cardiac evaluation of all patients over 70 years old and encouraged them to see a specific cardiologist who performed a more extensive evaluation including an electrocardiogram, echocardiogram, carotid and abdominal ultrasound, coronary computed tomography angiography, and occasionally a 3-day cardiac rhythm monitor. This program has reduced the cost of cardiac complications.

3.4 Florida Orthopaedic Institute Experience with BPCI 2 Risk Bundle Program

The Florida Orthopedic Institute was awarded participation in BPCI 2 to manage our primary hip and knee replacement patients and hip replacements for hip fracture between January 2015 and September 2018. 3186 total hip and knee replacements were enrolled in this program.

We were able to achieve a 17% reduction in hospital costs and a 9.2% reduction in hospital readmissions. However, the majority of savings were achieved from reductions in postoperative rehabilitation. There was a 5% reduction in inpatient rehabilitation stays. The largest savings occurred with skilled nursing facilities with a 12% reduction in admissions (Fig. 3.1) and 34% reduced length of stay (Fig. 3.2). The percentage admissions to home health care was unchanged, but there was a 35% reduction in average visits (Fig. 3.3). Twelve percent more patients were sent to outpatient physical therapy, but the total outpatient physical therapy visits were unchanged.

We were able to provide an average per patient savings to Medicare of $1793 which equates to an estimated total savings on our 3186 patients of $5,700,000. The liaison between our group and CMS received 35% of the savings. The remaining savings went to pay for case manager salaries, expenses, waiver costs, the operating surgeon, and the remainder to the group. The maximum gain share to the operating surgeon was capped at 60% which amounted to an approximate 8% bonus over the standard Medicare reimbursement. The remainder of the savings went to the orthopedic group.

Some non-modifiable high-risk patients have not undergone surgical intervention. Either their risk for a complication or readmission or the requirement to assume financial responsibility for the costs of other ongoing medical treatments during the episode of care were deemed too high.

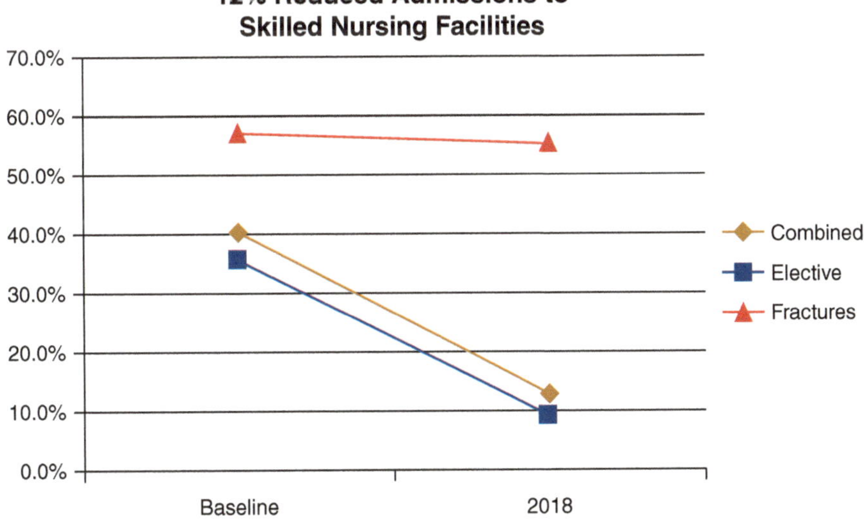

Fig. 3.1 Reduced admissions to skilled nursing facilities

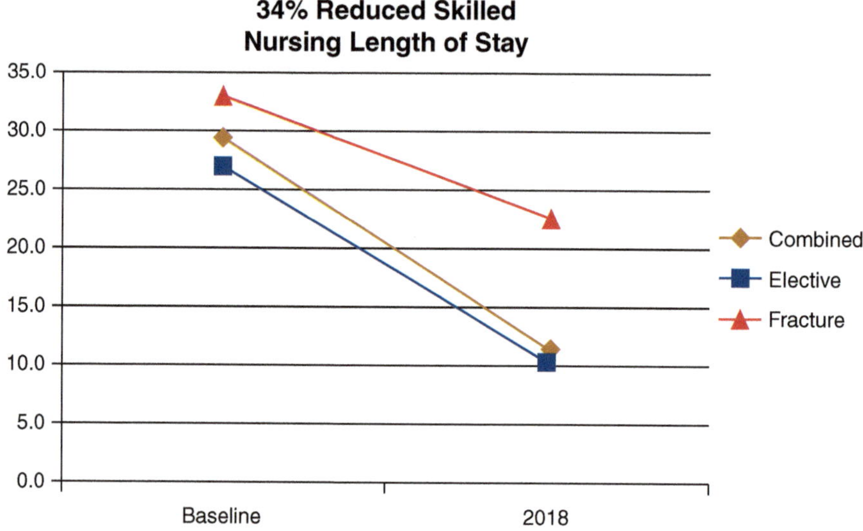

Fig. 3.2 Reduced skilled nursing length of stay

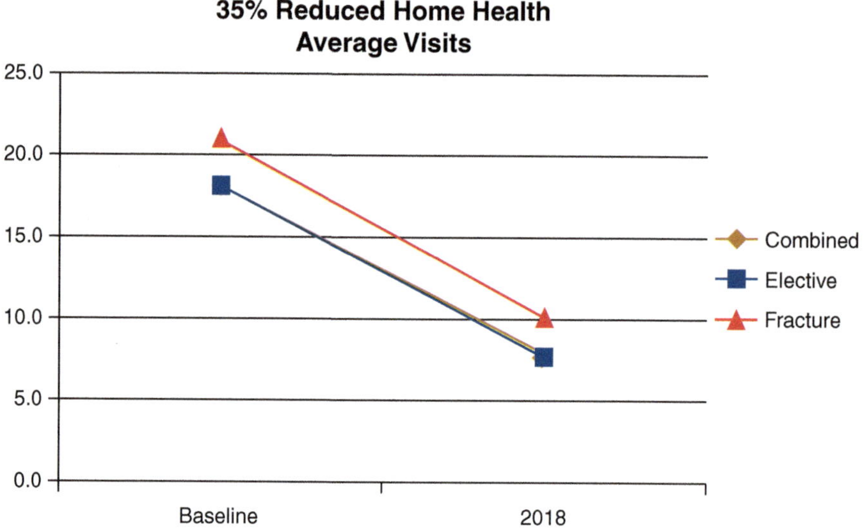

Fig. 3.3 Reduced home health average visits

3.5 Summary

CMS's goal to reduce overall cost was significantly achieved. We were still able to improve patient outcomes by an increased effort to optimize patients medically prior to surgery. We have seen the benefit of taking more control over the pre-operative evaluation and medical clearance and the benefit of developing relationships with cardiologists in the optimization of patients. Relationships with specific skilled nursing facilities and home health agencies were developed to have direct control of all post-discharge rehabilitation. The patients were able to spend more time at home rather than in skilled nursing facilities during recovery. Case managers were hired to assist in developing the post-discharge plan and continue throughout the episode of care with communication with the patient and rehab providers.

The orthopedic provider has benefited by an additional reimbursement bonus per case. Participation in this program required a great amount of time spent by the physicians, physician extenders, and case managers in developing the initial program, for which the arthroplasty physicians were not directly reimbursed by the group outside of the average 8% increased reimbursement per case. If one considers the estimated 50+ hours spent by each of the surgeons in meetings in establishing and monitoring the program, the bonuses are not as significant. However, knowledge was gained in how to successfully manage a care bundle. As other orthopedic procedures have been brought into bundled programs, reduced time has been necessary for other orthopedic surgeons in our group to ramp up their programs. Now that we have demonstrated the ability to successfully manage the program, we probably have less need for the conveners.

The additional organization costs to manage the bundle may be cost prohibitive for most individual or small physician groups. Since savings were compared to historic costs, those providers with higher historic costs could see the greatest financial benefit. However, subsequent BPCI programs have reset the historic cost target, thereby reducing the potential for further cost savings and incentive for providers to participate. One gets the feeling that these programs could be a "race to the bottom" for reimbursement for patient care. This would result in only cherry-picking low-risk patients for care.

Not every patient who would benefit from hip or knee arthroplasty was able to be optimized medically in order to decrease the risk for complications or readmission. There needs to be risk-adjustments developed for patients with higher or non-modifiable comorbidities and lower socioeconomic status so that access to care is not affected.

The BPCI bundle programs have ended for hip and knee joint replacement. We are participating in a hospital managed Comprehensive Care for Joint Replacement Model (CJR) bundle. Because the savings are not as high, CMS will probably again encourage physician ownership of bundles because we have more control over the post-discharge spend.

We feel strongly that in order for these programs to be successful in the future, physicians deserve to "sit at the table" to help develop future programs with fair benchmarks and have the option to continue to manage the programs. Physicians understand the need to control costs but are still the patient's advocate for quality care.

References

1. Hawker GA, Badley EM, Croxford R, et al. A population-based nested case-control study of the costs of hip and knee replacement surgery. Med Care. 2009;47:732–41.
2. Clair AJ, Evangelista PJ, Lajam CM, et al. Cost analysis of total joint arthroplasty readmissions in a bundled payment care improvement initiative. J Arthroplast. 2016;31:1862–5.
3. Althausen PL, Mead L. Bundled payments for care improvement: lessons learned in the first year. J Orthop Trauma. 2016;Suppl 5:50–3.
4. Cutler DM, Ghosh K. The potential for cost savings through bundled episode payments. N Engl J Med. 2012;366:1075–7.
5. Manickas-Hill O, Feeley T, Bozic KJ. A review of bundled payments in total joint replacement. J Bone Joint Surg Rev. 2019;7:1–7.
6. Siddiqi A, White PB, Mistry JB, et al. Effect of bundled payments and health care reform as alternative payment models in total joint arthroplasty: a clinical review. J Arthroplast. 2017;32:2590–7.
7. Iorio R, Clair AJ, Inneh IA, et al. Early results of Medicare's bundled payment initiative for a 90-day total joint arthroplasty episode of care. J Arthroplast. 2016;31:343–50.
8. Iorio R. Strategies and tactics for successful implementation of bundled payments: bundled payment for care improvement at a large, urban, academic medical center. J Arthroplast. 2015;30:349–50.
9. Courtney PM, Huddleston JL, Iorio R, Markel DC. Socioeconomic risk adjustments models for reimbursement are necessary in primary total joint arthroplasty. J Arthroplast. 2017;32:1–5.

Latest Advances in Cardiac Imaging Modalities

4

Nghia H. Ho and Eric E. Harrison

Abstract

Current advancements and evolution of medical knowledge and technology in medical imaging devices have improved image quality and reduced the need for invasive procedures to patients. Modern-day medical machines, such as Computed Tomography (CT) and Magnetic Resonance Imaging (MRI), have paved the way for the evolution of cardiac scanning from CT Coronary Angiography (CCTA), Cardiac MRI (CMR), and Cardiac Positron Emission Tomography (PET)/CT Imaging. Along with advancements in 4D-strain echocardiography, these new advancements are proven aids in providing quicker and more accurate evaluations of cardiac morphology, functionality, and risks over the legacy modalities, such as the spectrum of stress tests and 2D, M-mode echocardiography of yesteryear. The techniques using modern imaging modalities continue to significantly improve the landscape of noninvasive diagnostic cardiology, resulting in significant leaps forward for medicine. These advancements are becoming more prevalent with the goal of increasing the accuracy of determining which patients will require invasive revascularization procedures and assessment tests and, ultimately, to achieve better outcomes while decreasing healthcare costs.

N. H. Ho
Midwestern University, Glendale, AZ, USA

Chicago State University, Chicago, IL, USA

PEPID, LLC, Tampa, FL, USA

E. E. Harrison (✉)
Board Chair International Cardio-Oncology Society,
ICOS CEO PrivaCors Inc. Cardio-Orthopaedics®, Tampa, FL, USA

Morsani College of Medicine, University of South Florida, Tampa, FL, USA

Joint Special Operations University, Tampa, FL, USA

E. E. Harrison, N. H. Ho (eds.), *Managing Cardiovascular Risk In Elective Total Joint Arthroplasty*, https://doi.org/10.1007/978-3-031-26415-3_4

Keywords

Coronary Computed Tomography Angiography (CCTA) · Cardiac MRI (CMR) · Cardiac Computed Tomography (CT) · Coronary artery disease · Fractional flow reserve (FFR) · CT-derived FFR · CT Coronary angiography (CTCA) · Cardiovascular disease risk · Cardiac PET/CT · 4D-strain echocardiography · Nuclear Single Photon Emissions CT scan (SPECT) · 2D and M-mode echocardiography · Cardiac stress tests · Magnetic resonance imaging (MRI) · Electrocardiogram (ECG) · ElektroKardioGraph (EKG)

Chapter Objectives

1. Case study presentation
2. Introduction to cardiac CT advancements
3. Introduction to perfusion PET/CT advancements
4. Introduction to cardiac MRI advancements
5. Introduction to 4D-strain echocardiography
6. Current disadvantages for patient care due to the persistence of legacy stress tests and 2D/M-mode echocardiography

4.1 Case Study Presentation

I was very excited about the development of a non-invasive modality to take the place of cardiac catheterization. Twenty thousand and three presented the opportunity with the first reports of the advances in 16 slice scanning to make a difference although there were certainly substantial developments to be had in the future to perfect this technology. But I saw this as an opportunity to make the move from diagnostic cardiac catheterization and stress tests to anatomical, functional, and morphological evaluation of heart disease where form follows function. I hung up my catheters and stents and also quite the current nuclear SPECT scanning that had been downgraded by radiology to no longer have a separate cardiac nuclear technologist to guide the complex technology. I would move into CCTA, PET/CT, and cardiac MRI as my reinvention of myself.

What was the impact on orthopedics? Perhaps an early version of evolutionary cardio-orthopedics as cardiology started to change technically. As an early example, in 2006 when I saw a 58-year-old male who was being evaluated for knee replacement. He recently had a SPECT scan with a fixed detent in the anterior wall. What was the plan and what was the risk? This would have been my chance to do a cardiac catheterization as I had done 14,000 times in the past. Or how about the new technology with the 16 slice CCTA scanner where I was working daily?

The patient's weight was 260 pounds which added considerable graininess to the quality of the images. His heart rate averaged 63 with a range of 61–70 bpm. He received 100 cc of Optiray IV and 40 mg of Propranolol to slow his heartbeat. There was poor contrast resolution of his heart making it impossible to view the anterior wall defect. The aorta was dilated at 39.2 × 40.3 mm. Total calcium score was 262:

LM 4, RCA 1, LAD 212, and LCX 45. Seventy five percent of males have lower calcium scores at this age. The images of the coronaries show very focal positively remodeled nodular <15% and certainly less than 50% plaques in the LAD and LCX with excellent distal flow. The plaques in the main left and RCA were not seen.

It was concluded that the perfusion defect was not real without significant CAD and that he needed to be on a statin. He was low risk for his TKA. This looked like a better test in even a difficult patient with low scan slices than a catheterization with risk and expense. I knew there were better instruments in development and being tested. Let's hear about the course of this development from Dr. Nghia H. Ho, MD.

4.2 Introduction

Advanced cardiac imaging consists of coronary CT, cardiac PET/CT, cardiac MRI (CMR), and 4D/strain echocardiography. These modalities are the most technically advanced ways of defining, distinguishing, and demonstrating the anatomy and physiology of the heart, but are currently still slow to be implemented and integrated into daily cardiac practice, as opposed to existing and outdated modalities, such as 2D and m-mode echocardiography, the spectrum of cardiac stress tests, including Single Photon Emission Computed Tomography (SPECT) scanning. The difference, with a distinction is: the use of the new testing versus legacy testing modalities is analogous to comparing a 1979 rotary landline phone with a current-day smartphone. However, the choice for selecting the old modalities (e.g., 2D and m-mode echo, SPECT, stress tests) over the new ones (e.g., coronary CT, PET/CT, CMR) is usually based on trying to avoid the complexity of navigating the medical industrial complex.

4.3 Advancements in Cardiac Computed Tomography

Rapid technological advancements in cardiac CT have improved image quality and reduced radiation exposure to patients. Furthermore, key insights from large cohort trials have helped delineate cardiovascular disease risk as a function of overall coronary plaque burden and the morphological appearance of individual plaques. The advent of CT-derived fractional flow reserve promises to establish an anatomical and functional test within one modality. Recent data examining the short-term impact of CT-derived fractional flow reserve on downstream care and clinical outcomes have been published. In addition, machine learning is a concept that is being increasingly applied to diagnostic medicine.

Over the coming decade, machine learning will begin to be integrated into cardiac CT and will potentially make a tangible difference to how this modality evolves [1, 2]. Recent advances currently impact clinical care and potential future directions for this imaging modality [3]. CCTA using 4- and 16-slice scanners, however, lacked the sufficient robustness to be clinically useful the majority of the time. Hence, the 64-slice (and higher) CT technologies have been developed to increase spatial and temporal resolution, which not only has improved clinical reliability, but also allows for the evaluation of the entire clinically relevant coronary tree. Among patients in whom a decision had already been made to obtain CCTA, 64-slice CCTA was reliable for ruling out significant CAD in patients with stable and unstable anginal syndromes [4]. However, a positive 64-slice CCTA scan often overestimates the severity of atherosclerotic obstructions and requires further testing to guide patient management.

4.4 The Physics of Cardiac CT Improved

Recent advancements such as increased gantry spin times and fast single heartbeat scanning have dramatically improved and enhanced image resolution as well as scan times, thus decreasing radiation exposure during each scanning session of the patient. The increased gantry spin times have allowed single heartbeat whole heart scanning—the time required for one rotation of the X-ray tube is halved by adding a second X-ray tube, allowing for the single beat whole heart capture at a specific R-R interval. This technique shortens the time for patients to be in the X-ray tube and alleviates stitching artefacts since the whole image is captured in one sequence. However, heart rate control is essential for this process and patients' heart rates are usually reduced with medicines prior to the scanning procedure. Because of these recent advancements, several guidelines have now recommended CCTA as first-line screening protocol for assessing recent onset chest pain [2].

Since this modality has been added to standard of care, there have been fewer cardiovascular disease (CVD) deaths or non-fatal MIs (HR 0.59; 95% CI [0.41–0.84]; $p = 0.004$) in association with CCTA use [5]. This, along with the excellent diagnostic sensitivity, specificity, positive-predictive value, and negative-predictive value (94%, 97%, 87%, and 99%, respectively) for detecting significant coronary artery disease [6], will continue to enhance better patient outcomes within the increasing scope of precision medicine.

4.5 Plaque Analysis with Cardiac CT

Coronary CT angiography (CCTA) and fractional flow reserve CT, along with computational fluid dynamics equations, can aid in predicting the functional implications of coronary artery lesions within hours. In comparison to current invasive FFR studies (i.e., flow reserve with cardiac catheterization procedure) [7], CT-derived FFR can be achieved by sending images from the non-invasive CCTA to a vendor (e.g., HeartFlow in the UK) that will use state-of-the-art software to analyze and color-code fractional flow within the specified coronary artery tree(s) (see Figs. 4.1 and 4.2). As CCTA and CT-derived FFR continue to move medicine forward, several constraints will have to be solved. Firstly, overcoming the difficulties of attaining good image quality due to high heart rate, obese body habitus, poor contrast evolution, and artefacts due to patient movements. Secondly, the "FFR grey zone"

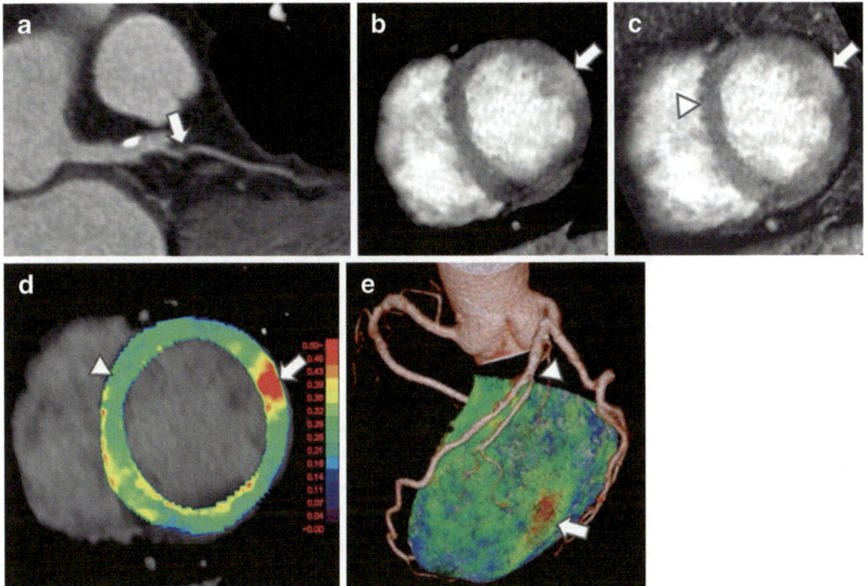

Fig. 4.1 Dual modality imaging pictures (**a**–**d**) with cardiac CTA with contrast and AI 3D rendering software (**e**)

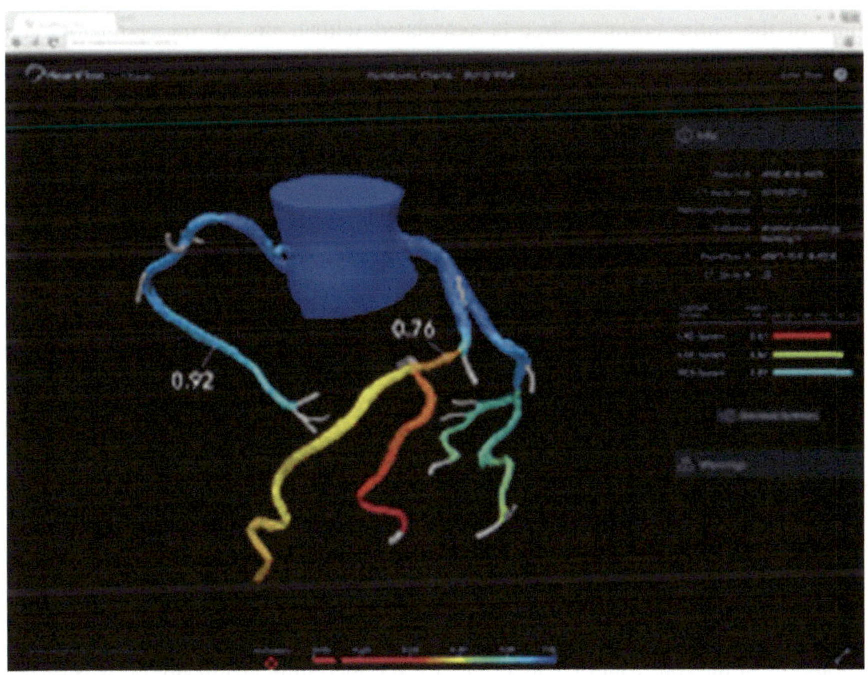

Fig. 4.2 AI CT FFR by heartflow

(i.e., CT-derived FFR 0.7–0.8) has negatively affected the diagnostic accuracy, reported in several studies (about 46% reviewed assessing 536 patients in total). Thirdly, there are no studies in post-revascularization patients. Finally, this computational service is limited to a single vendor (i.e., HeartFlow).

Another useful and practical aspect of CCTA is its ability to quantify the morphology of the plagues and lesions. In terms of plague assessment, CCTA has prospered due to recent work establishing the concept of vulnerable plague identification on CT, which can be used to confer risk for acute coronary syndrome. This showed that high-risk plaque composition (necrotic core to fibrous plaque ratio) correlates with fibroatheromas seen on intravascular ultrasound. CCTA can also be used to demonstrate positive remodeling as well as low-attenuation plaques being associated with fibroatheromas with macrophage infiltration. Thusly, vulnerable plaque detection by CCTA has been used as an indication for aggressive prevention strategies for patient care. CCTA together with flow assessment can also help to quantify the amount of stenosis, thereby, with semi-automatic scoring systems, can help with establishing markers, such as segmental stenosis score and segmental involvement score. These scores can then be used to quantify the burden of disease and aid in prognostication. With the additive ability of CCTA to be able to reveal the characteristics of individual plaques to diameter stenosis, improved predictability of functionally significant lesions can be determined.

In addition to revealing plaque morphology, CCTA can also demonstrate total plaque volume. This whole-vessel approach makes the evaluation of the coronary tree much more predictive of overall plaque burden. For example, total plaque volume of the entire coronary tree is associated with high risk for cardiac-related death [8].

Recent advancements in medical software AI algorithm studies have shown even more usefulness of CCTA scanning. With implementing the same CCTA scans from any single session, not only can the internal morphology of coronary arteries be evaluated, as aforementioned, but the external surface morphology of the coronaries can also be examined as to the inflammatory affects and consequences that the visceral fat layers have on the coronary arteries. It is now possible to calculate the risk for having a major adverse cardiac event from a CCTA scan by calculating its Fat Attenuation Index scores. Furthermore, other medical software AIs are currently underway to combine such algorithms to produce more diagnostic computations that can advance CCTA scan usefulness.

4.6 Machine Learning

With the advent of recent technologies and the ongoing evolution of techno-medical fusion, machine learning for healthcare providers is becoming more vital to the standard of care for patients. With computer-based algorithms increasingly being applied to clinical imaging to aid in medical decision-making, machine learning should be at the forefront of importance for the incoming healthcare professionals. The cornerstone of machine learning is its ability to analyze large data sets to extract what data is applicable to predict potential clinically significant lesions in order to improve diagnoses and outcomes. It can also quantify markers that can enter into scoring systems. Machine learning, along with CCTA data sets, has shown to be superior in detecting ischemic lesions by calculating CT perfusion and adding it to the severity of stenosis.

The integration of machine learning with CCTA continues to provide exciting opportunities to aid the physician with predicting risk for the patient. As these integrations become more relevant in the medical world, the scope of machine learning will continue to grow. The potential benefits from this integration, such as improved precision of diagnoses and ischemia detection, enhanced risk prediction, and reduced healthcare costs, will soon usher in a better way to provide more effective healthcare to patients.

4.7 Advancements in Cardiac PET/CT

The non-invasive, hybrid imaging technique of positron emission tomography (PET) with computed tomography (CT) has become an important, key modality for precision medical imaging and evaluation in cardiology [9]. It allows for the quantification of cardiac perfusion as well as anatomical mapping of the coronary arteries, accurate assessments that can be done in less than an hour per scanning session. This method can provide a wealth of much needed information for (suspected) coronary artery disease (CAD). In eventuality, this novel hybrid imaging method can guide clinical patient management and effect a higher rate of positive outcomes. Cardiac PET continues to improve the understanding of the pathophysiological processes and functionality of the coronary vasomotor system. It has also proven to be greater in diagnostic accuracy in detecting obstruction in coronary artery disease than Single Photon Emission Computed Tomography (SPECT) [10, 11].

Even with these clear advantages, cardiac PET currently is not as prevalent as its more available and lesser costly modalities. However, the recent combination of PET scanning with CT imaging to form the PET/CT hybrid modality has been gaining popularity, especially in the realms of clinical oncology and cardiology, and has led to its world-wide growth. This growth has coincided with the expansion of cardiac CT scanning applications, such as coronary artery calcium scoring and contrast CT coronary angiography. The ability of cardiac PET/CT to aid in the evaluation of the anatomy, morphology, and functionality of the coronary arteries in one scan practically in real-time has shown a positive transformation in the clinical management of patients with or suspected for coronary artery disease.

4.7.1 Physics of PET

PET scanning uses artificially produced radionuclides (tracers) that emit positive-charged particles (positrons) that are inhaled, ingested, or injected into the body, depending on what tissue(s) or system(s) being evaluated. Once the positrons travel through the tissue(s) (in millimeters), they collide and annihilate with an electron, thus producing two photons that disperse in opposite vectors (line of response), which are then detected and recorded by the PET scanner (in nanoseconds) [9–11]. The recording of all the lines of response then form a 3-D map of the structures being evaluated.

4.7.2 SPECT vs PET/CT

Some of the issues that give PET/CT hybrid imaging advantages over SPECT are noted to be its accuracy, resolution, time of results, and radiation exposure risks. Attenuation artifacts can be reduced with the use of the CT, reducing the false-positive perfusion defects, leading to increased specificity and, thus, accuracy. Also, the higher resolution of PET (5–7 mm) than SPECT (about 15 mm) further enhances PET imaging accuracy by reducing the false-negative results. Furthermore, PET perfusion tracer extraction fraction is higher than SPECT, which allows PET to detect more subtle perfusion differences otherwise missed with SPECT scanning.

Another advantageous aspect of PET/CT over SPECT is its lower radiation exposure risks. This is due to the shorter physical half-life and low radiation burden of the PET tracers (less than 10 mSv) compared with the SPECT tracers (greater than 10 mSv), as well as the ability of PET/CT scanning to acquire both rest and stress images in a single scanning session (in contrast with multiple-day sessions for SPECT protocol) [9]. Finally, the short resolution duration of the radioactive tracers in PET (in seconds) allows for measurements of perfusion in mL per minute per gram of tissue for the quantification of regional Myocardial Blood Flow (rMBF). This provides both a qualitative myocardial perfusion image and absolute levels of perfusion and flow reserve measurements.

4.7.3 Diagnostic Accuracy of PET and its Radionuclides (Tracers)

Perfusion PET positron emitting tracers most commonly used are $H_2{}^{15}O$, $^{13}NH_3$, and Rubidium. $H_2{}^{15}O$ is metabolically inert, freely diffusible, and not affected by flow-dependent extraction rates; thus, its complete myocardial extraction from arterial blood makes this tracer ideal to quantify perfusion. However, it may provide very little diagnostic value as it yields low signal gradients between compartments; hence, it is usually not used clinically. $^{13}NH_3$ and Rubidium are actively trapped in the myocardial tissue and produce high quality myocardial perfusion images (MPI). However, because they have incomplete, non-linear extraction at increasing flow rates, this results in less accurate quantification of perfusion.

Due to the very short half-life and deep positron emission tissue penetration depth, Rubidium is considered the least accurate tracer in comparison with $H_2{}^{15}O$ and $^{13}NH_3$. Rubidium also requires and expensive on-site cyclotron to generate. The most commonly used tracers in studies on diagnostic accuracy of myocardial perfusion imaging with PET for the detection of obstructive CAD have been $^{13}NH_3$ and Rubidium.

4.7.4 Accuracy of Perfusion PET

Recent studies have been reviewed to show the weighted specificity to be 89% and the sensitivity to be 90% with diagnostic accuracy of PET (analyzed from multiple studies including 877 patients) [10]. Comparison studies of SPECT with PET accuracy have consistently shown PET to be superior, with increased sensitivity of 91% with $^{13}NH_3$ (PET) vs. 81% with Thallium-201 (SPECT) tracers and 93% specificity with Rubidium (PET) vs. 85% with Thallium-201 (SPECT) [12]. Another study also compared PET with SPECT using ^{99}T-sestamibi, which also resulted in a higher specificity with PET (93% vs 73%, respectively), as well as a higher sensitivity with PET (87% vs 82%, respectively) [13].

As for prognostication studies, SPECT has had well defined and long-term follow-up of large cohorts of CAD patients. However, the relatively newer perfusion PET scan procedure has recently gained greater popularity and also is becoming more established. For example, a large cohort study of 685 patients showing the prognostic implications of relative MPI with Rubidium PET resulted in an event-free survival after a 41-month follow-up of 90% normal scan, 87% mildly abnormal scan, 75% moderately abnormal scan, and 76% extensively abnormal scan [14]. Additionally, the absolute quantitative flow prognostic value was studied in ischemic heart disease patients. This study showed, of 344 patients using $^{13}NH_3$ PET, increased mortality was independently related to the level of flow reserve impairment and that it was a stronger predictor of cardiac death than left ventricular ejection fraction [14]. Other studies have also shown the prognostic value with Rubidium PET scanning [15], and more studies with larger cohorts continue to establish the superiority of PET over SPECT.

4.7.5 Combining PET and CT Imaging in CAD Patients

Recent innovations and continuing technical progress with cardiac CTA as a standalone scan has validated it as a valuable tool in the assessment of CAD patients. As an initial screening tool, it is currently well established that a normal cardiac CT can accurately rule out CAD. However, low quality scans or scans showing coronary lesions will require additional testing to establish accurate prognosis. It is clear that, due to the increased false-positive results from either CT or PET MPI alone, it can lead to missed diagnoses and unnecessary invasive procedures. However, with the hybridization of both PET and CT, combining the two complementary information from a single hour-long session, all the required and actionable data can be attained to guide patient management decision-making (Fig. 4.3). For example, a normal CT and PET MPI rules out CAD in the patient, which can be an indication for patient discharge (see Fig. 4.1).

Furthermore, CCTA and perfusion PET together can also help pinpoint coronary lesions that produce ischemia by combining both the anatomical and functional images, thereby identifying the location of the obstruction in question which can aid in employing correct percutaneous treatment strategies [16]. Also, if there are no

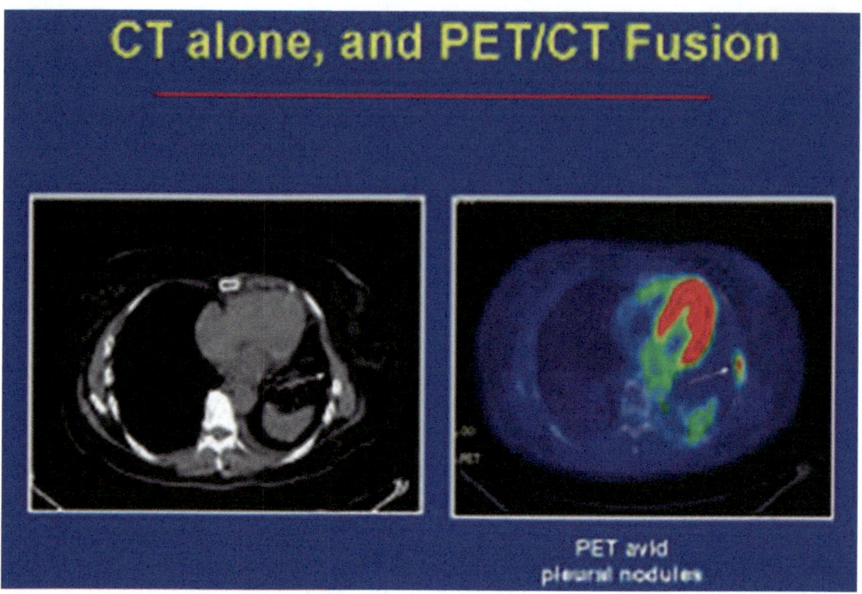

Fig. 4.3 CT alone vs PET/CT

signs of epicardial coronary artery lesions and yet show regional perfusion defects or flow impairment, it is reasonable to conclude microvascular dysfunction in the coronary artery.

4.8 Advancements in Cardiac Magnetic Resonance Imaging

Cardiac magnetic resonance (CMR) imaging has been proven to provide accurate information of the anatomy of the heart, its vasculature, and advanced soft contrast. Thus, CMR is currently the reference standard for evaluating cardiac volumes and systolic function pathologies. New advancements and achievements in technical development has made CMR imaging more prevalent and has broadened it beyond its use just for characterizing myocardial lesions or contractility evaluations. CMR sequences can now offer more comprehensive diagnostic evaluations of myocardial tissue fiber orientation, coronary plaque characteristics, and metabolic activity. At the same time, it can make these diagnostic data available almost immediately to be applied towards patient care decision-making in the clinical setting [17].

With all these potentially excellent benefits, CMR, however, currently has several limitations, including its high cost, time-consuming procedure, and limited availability. Optimistically, recent technological advances in software and hardware are driving CMR utility in cardiology towards new heights.

4.8.1 Physics of Cardiac Magnetic Resonance Imaging

With the production of high quality, accurate imaging of anatomical information and its advanced soft contrast abilities, CMR has shown to be superior over other imaging modalities in its ability to discriminate cardiac lesions. It is the cardiac imaging reference standard today for quantifying morphology of cardiac chambers and cardiac systolic function. It can also provide practical and diagnostic insight into the pathological and physiological progression of disease of the cardiac tissues with its myocardium characterization techniques, which include T1-, T2-, T2-star weighted mapping, and late gadolinium enhancement (LGE) functions. With the introduction of 3 T MRI as another function, which has significantly improved spatial resolution and diagnostic accuracy in assessing the heart and its coronary vasculature, CMR imaging is becoming more routinely indicated for the evaluation of cardiac patients with various cardiomyopathies and coronary artery diseases.

Native T1 value (assessed with T1-mapping) is a composition of signals from myocytes and extracellular volume. An advantage it has over other modes is it does not require gadolinium-based contrast. Thus, can be used in patients with kidney comorbidities. Non-contrast T1 is most useful in detecting and demonstrating myocardial edema, diffuse interstitial fibrosis, and myocardium deposition of proteins and other substances (e.g., lipids, iron). When the native T1 value increases, this is indicative of disorders and diseases that cause myocardial edema, such as acute MI. Increasing native T1 value can also be due to an increase in interstitial space, which can be seen in interstitial fibrosis as a result of infarction or other cardiomyopathies. If the native T1 value is decreased, this can be due to lipid or iron overload disorders [18]. Gadolinium-enhanced contrast T1 mapping is used with extracellular volume expansion calculations. Extracellular volume is a marker for myocardial remodeling, and its expansion is a hallmark for heart failure. As the contrast perfuses the interstitial space, it shortens the T1 relaxation times proportional to the local concentration of gadolinium. This means that myocardial areas that are fibrosed or have scar tissue show shorter T1 relaxation times once the contrast is given. Increased extracellular volume (normal values have been shown to be 25.3 ± 3.5% [19]) is usually due to collagen deposition (i.e., fibrosis), while reduced extracellular volume is a result of lipomatous metaplasia or thrombus. Recently, uses for T1 and extracellular volume calculations can be helpful as an important tool for prognostication of CAD patients as well as evaluating non-ischemic cardiomyopathies. For example, native T1 accurately discriminates between normal hearts, hypertrophic cardiomyopathy, and heart disease due to hypertension [20, 21].

T2-weighted mapping is used to accurately pinpoint areas of myocardial edema due to acute inflammation. Hence, it can be useful in assessing acute myocardial infarction, myocarditis, stress cardiomyopathy, and even heart allograft rejection. T2-STIR is also commonly used to distinguish between acute and chronic infarctions although T2 mapping is more reproducible and can be quantified directly in vivo [22]. Also, T2 mapping was superior when compared to T1 mapping and extracellular volume for evaluating myocarditis in recent-onset heart failure with reduced ejection fraction [23]. As CMR technology progresses, we may even see more and more, multitasking integrations, where CMR software can enable T1, T1/T2, and time-resolved T1 mappings to be done simultaneously. This ability for CMR to capture images continuously in multiple mapping techniques would allow for conceptualization of the physiologic motions of the heart and its processes in multiple time dimensions, thus, making it possible to have efficient quantitative CMR imaging without breath holds and ECG gating.

Late-gadolinium enhancement (LGE) is a T1-weighted technique that allows for the detection and quantification of myocardium injury and infiltration in cardiac diseases. It is currently the gold standard technique for identifying myocardial scar tissue. This technique calculates the velocity and pattern of contrast distribution and accumulation in the myocardium extracellular compartment. This pattern reflects the disease process and progression of myocardial damage, and, thus, identifies the etiology of the disease. For example, as the pattern of progression for ischemia in CAD patients occur from subendocardial tissue with transmural extension, the LGE pattern will follow this process, whereas, in dilated cardiomyopathy, the LGE will be a more linear mid-wall pattern in distribution within the interventricular septum [24]. Furthermore, another benefit for the LGE technique that has significance with guiding clinical decision-making is its ability to delineate myocardial tissue viability in both ischemic and non-ischemic cardiac diseases. However, some limiting factors for LGE use are its limited ability to assess early cardiac disease changes, as well as limited scope of utility because it is useful mainly for cardiac diseases that results in regional differences in the myocardium [25]. Further CMR advancements look into assessments of myocardial fiber orientation with diffusion tensor imaging (DTI) and myocardial metabolic activity (for additional information of the fiber viability characterizations and assessment and understanding of the pathophysiology of disease progression, respectively) [26].

4.8.2 Coronary Artery Plaque Imaging

As the preference for choice of modality for coronary angiography is shifting from invasive to non-invasive procedures, there is a growing need for evaluating CAD with non-invasive methods, such as CCTA and coronary magnetic resonance angiography (MRA). Some advantages of coronary MRA, which can potentially make it an invaluable complementary imaging modality for longitudinal studies, include superior soft-tissue contrast allowing for better characterization of high-risk plaques, the fact that coronary MRA does not expose the patients to radiation, and the absence of blooming artifacts which can make assessments of the lumen of severely calcified vessels possible and clearer than CCTA [27]. However, coronary MRA is lagging due to the small size and complex movements of these vessels, which is better captured with CCTA than coronary MRA.

4.9 Advancements in 4D: Strain Echocardiography

4D-strain echocardiography is gaining widespread acceptance at clinical institutions for its high temporal resolution and relatively low cost [28]. As the leading cause of death in the United States, the ability for doctors to be able to understand more fully and have the appropriate tools to diagnose heart disease pathologies early equates to better outcomes and can begin to flatten the upward trend of this statistical and literal nightmare for so many patients and their families. The technique of 4D echocardiography imaging has the ability to recover and demonstrate dense myocardial displacement, thereby helping doctors better diagnose such maladies. This technology not only can show more precise results, but also aid in training and teaching future physicians with more accurate and clear imaging standards of the cardiac structures and progression of pathology on these structures.

Myocardial strain obtained from displacement vectors with 4D echocardiography technique can also play a vital role in assisting with more accurate diagnosing of cardiac disorders [29]. First defined in 2D echocardiography imaging in 1973, strain at that time represented systolic deformation occurring after the application of stress [30]. Strain is given by the following formula:

$$\varepsilon = \frac{L - L_0}{L_0} = \frac{\Delta L}{\Delta L_0}$$

Strain is ε, L_0 is the baseline length of the myocardium, and L is the length after systolic deformation. The strain, defined as fractional length change in one dimension, is expressed in (%) units of positive (lengthening of myocardium) or negative (shortening of myocardium) [31]. While this technique and calculation was a necessary step in the right direction for the evolution of cardiology, it is necessary to also remember that the heart is a 3D organ whose structure and function has by now been demonstrated with complex fiber arrangements. Hence, when applying strain imaging, it is vital that there are three main spatial orientations (vectors) associated with the left ventricular myocardial contraction to be demonstrated in order to be more accurate.

The first special orientation is the longitudinal aspect, which occurs from base to apex as the mitral annulus contracts towards the left ventricular apex (a negative strain occurs as systolic contraction towards the ensonifying transducer located at the apex from the traditional four-chamber apical view). Contrastingly, as the oblique fibers of the myocardium are seen from the short axis view, based on the myocardial band arrangement, then two forms of contraction would be seen as resulting in myocardial thickening, recently characterized as the "twisting motion" of the myocardium. The second orientation involves the radial contraction (or relative thickening) of the left ventricular wall towards the center, which results in a positive strain. The third orientation is the counterclockwise-clockwise motion of the myocardial fibers seen from base-to-apex and from apex-to-base, respectively.

This motion during systole, characterized as the "wringing motion," effectively reduces the left ventricular cavity size (circumferential shortening) and is seen as negative strain. It is important to note that during diastole the left ventricle relaxes as it returns to its resting state and the myocardial motion would be in the opposite direction from systole; hence, the strain designation would also follow suit (i.e., if systolic strain is positive, then diastolic strain would be negative). This difference between the basal and apical segments strain is the "rotation" expressed in degrees per second. The rate of strain, the rate of deformation (i.e., stretch) over time, can be calculated from the following equation:

$$\varepsilon = \frac{\Delta\varepsilon}{\Delta t} = \frac{(\Delta L / \Delta L\mathrm{o})}{\Delta t} = \frac{(\Delta L / \Delta t)}{\mathrm{Lo}} = \frac{\Delta V}{\mathrm{Lo}}$$

The velocity gradient of the segment is ΔV. Both the strain and rate of strain are in the same direction. It is also important to note that this deformation does not directly measure myocardial contractility, which represents the active state of the myocardium (i.e., strain is a load-dependent measurement).

In order to characterize complex, rapidly moving cardiac structures, high spatial and temporal resolution data is a requirement. 4D-strain echocardiography is one of the few modalities that can achieve this with minimal risks and cost when compared to other modalities, such as fluoroscopy, X-ray CT, or MRI. However, modern 4D-strain echocardiography imaging is still affected by noise and artifacts, which makes analyzing the data difficult, even though there has been great progress made in the development of piezoelectric elements and signal processing techniques. Hence, 4D-strain echocardiography algorithms are still being developed to better cope with these artifacts.

4.9.1 Experience

Within the medical industrial complex, challenges of implementing and integrating modern cardiac technologies have to deal with resistance to knowledge and training acquisition. While cardiologists understand and know the majority of the organ knowledge, at least 80%, they must undergo training to understand the minimal 20% of technical know-how required to achieve expertise in use of and diagnosing with these advanced imaging modalities (which is extremely "do-able"). On the other hand, there is also resistance from radiologists, who have been taking a piece of the financial pie, who would rather continue doing what they have been doing and not move on to such new, more accurate, and less cost-enticing modalities. While they (radiologists) already know the 20% unknown to cardiologists, they would have to learn the more than 80% vast knowledge of cardiology (which is extremely difficult) (see Fig. 4.4).

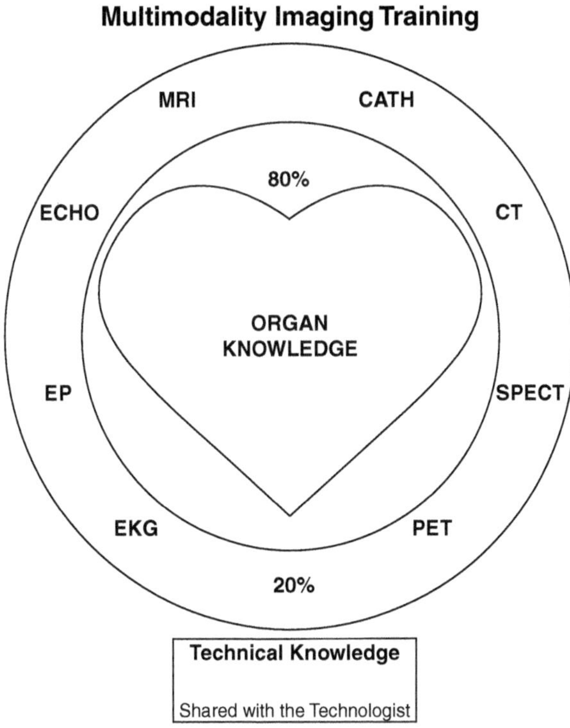

Fig. 4.4 Cardiologists know 80% of the organ knowledge and would have to learn 20% of the technical knowledge, whereas radiologists know the 20% of the technical knowledge and would have to learn an impossible 80% of the organ knowledge. Figure: Multimodality imaging training

4.10 Accuracy vs Cost

Since the development of echocardiography by Swedish physician Inge Edler in 1911, US accrediting bodies founded in the 1970s have continued to make old technologies like 2D and M-mode echocardiography mainstays of medical diagnostic tools. However, with the myriad of studies having shown the superior advantages of modern technological advances in precision cardiac imaging tools aforementioned, the stubborn, slow moving medical industrial complex giant still clings on to the highly inaccurate but financially lucrative revenue creating 1970s tools.

In one study, 81% of the abnormal tests were confirmed to be false positives. In this cohort, exercise stress test had a sensitivity of 0% for MI, a false-positive rate over 80%, and probably resulted in unnecessary invasive procedures [32]. In another study, the false-positive rate was between 58% and 100% [33]. Even with more studies done over the years, such as the Kahre (2008) study, which showed 64% of patients with positive stress tests were actually negative (false positive) when angiogram was done unnecessarily (based on cardiac stress test positive results), they were still performed to the detriment of the patients' pocketbooks, to the costs for the patients with positive stress tests being five times higher than those with negative stress tests. What do all of these widely inaccurate studies show regarding stress testing (without or without 2D echo)? In other words, stress testing had a sensitivity of 0% and a specificity of 0% [34]. In fact, of those cardiac stress tested that were normal, at least 40% will be false negative. Meaning, 4 out of 10 patients who truly need definitive treatment will not get it because the cardiac stress test reported inaccurate positive results. Also, of those having been cardiac stress tested, at least 65% will have false positive and have to endure unnecessary invasive procedures while accruing higher medical expenses. (Harrison)

4.11 Chapter Summary

In review, it is vitally important that as technology and medical societies continue towards better understanding of advances in software and hardware, doctors and hospitals should also continue to accept, procure, and evolve with these technologies. In doing so, push forward towards less invasive and more accurate diagnostic imaging results. With that will also come better medical decision-making and, ultimately, better outcomes and more cost-effective strategies for our patients.

With such precision technological advancements like CMR, CCTA, and 4D-Strain Echo, one would think the medical industrial complex would reach forth and grab hold of such incredible diagnostic tools to ensure a brighter future with better, more precise imaging techniques that cause much less harm to the patients (see Fig. 4.5). Yet, the seemingly myriad hurdles that has to be overcome can seem

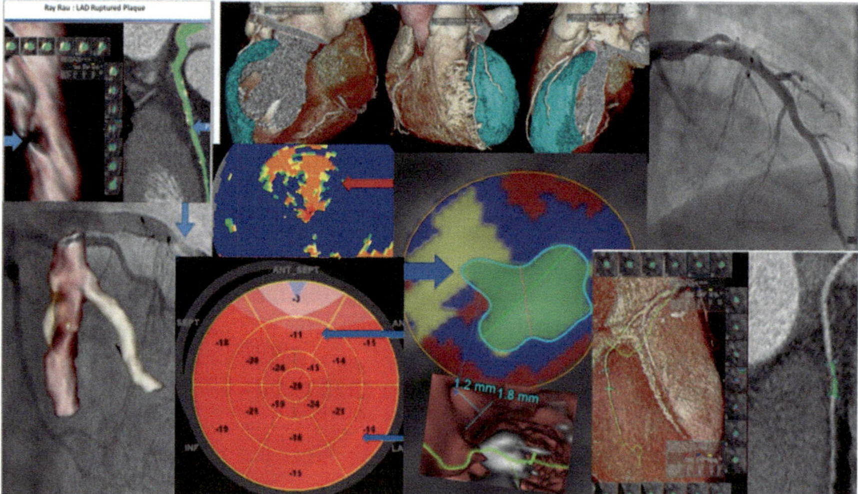

Fig. 4.5 Applied concomitant use of AI applications with multimodality analysis can be a more accurate function and produce higher yield accurate information than any single imaging source alone

overwhelming, but basically, comes down to revenue vs costs vs inexperience and the slow-moving conservatism of the medical industrial complex itself. Truly, one could expound on the saying, "tell me what year they graduated medical school, and I will tell you how they practice medicine."

References

1. Heseltine TD, Murray SW, Ruzsics B, Fisher M. Latest advances in cardiac CT. Eur Cardiology Rev. 2020;15:1.
2. Kelion AD, Nicol ED. The rationale for the primacy of coronary CT angiography in the National Institute for health and care excellence (NICE) guideline (CG95) for the investigation of chest pain of recent onset. J Cardiovasc Comput Tomogr. 2018;112:516–22.
3. British Society of Cardiovascular Imaging, Royal College of Radiologists. Fatal heart conditions going undetected due to lack of scanning services. 2018. https://bsci.org.uk/wp-content/uploads/2019/01/idor_2018_uk_release.pdf. Accessed 18 Dec 2019.
4. Meijboom WB, Meijs MFL, Schuijf JD, et al. Diagnostic accuracy of 64-slice computed tomography coronary angiography. A prospective, multicenter, multivendor study. J Am Coll Cardiol. 2008;52:2135–44.
5. SCOT-HEART Investigators. Coronary CT angiography and 5-year risk of myocardial infarction. N Engl J Med. 2018;379:924–33. https://doi.org/10.1056/NEJMoa1805971.
6. Ramjattan NA, Lala V, Kousa O, et al. Coronary CT angiography. In: StatPearls. Treasure Island (FL): StatPearls Publishing; 2020.
7. Renard BM, Cami E, Jiddou-Patros MR, et al. Optimizing the technique for invasive fractional flow reserve to assess lesion-specific ischemia. Circulation. 2019;12(10):e007939. https://doi.org/10.1161/CIRCINTERVENTIONS.119.007939.
8. Hell MM, Motwani M, Otaki Y, et al. Quantitative global plaque characteristics from coronary computed tomography angiography for the prediction of future cardiac mortality during long-term follow-up. Eur Heart J Cardiovasc Imaging. 2017;18:1331–9. https://doi.org/10.1093/ehjci/jex183.
9. Knaapen P, de Haan S, Hoekstra OS, et al. Cardiac PET-CT: advanced hybrid imaging for the detection of coronary artery disease. Neth Heart J. 2010;18(2):90–8. https://doi.org/10.1007/BF03091744.
10. Di Carli MF, Hachamovitch R. New technology for noninvasive evaluation of coronary artery disease. Circulation. 2007;115:1464–80. https://doi.org/10.1161/CIRCULATIONAHA.106.629808.
11. Le Guludec D, Lautamaki R, Knuuti J, Bax JJ, Bengel FM. Present and future of clinical cardiovascular PET imaging in Europe—a position statement by the European Council of Nuclear Cardiology (ECNC). Eur J Nucl Med Mol Imaging. 2008;35:1709–24. https://doi.org/10.1007/s00259-008-0859-1.
12. Machac J. Cardiac positron emission tomography imaging. Semin Nucl Med. 2005;35:17–36. https://doi.org/10.1053/j.semnuclmed.2004.09.002.
13. Bateman TM, Heller GV, McGhie AI, et al. Diagnostic accuracy of rest/stress ECG-gated Rb-82 myocardial perfusion PET: comparison with ECG gated Tc-99m sestamibi SPECT. J Nucl Cardiol. 2006;13:24–33. https://doi.org/10.1016/j.nuclcard.2005.12.004.
14. Marwick TH, Shan K, Patel S, Go RT, Lauer MS. Incremental value of rubidium-82 positron emission tomography for prognostic assessment of known or suspected coronary artery disease. Am J Cardiol. 1997;80:865–70. https://doi.org/10.1016/S0002-9149(97)00537-7.
15. Tio RA, Dabeshlim A, Siebelink HM, et al. Comparison between the prognostic value of left ventricular function and myocardial perfusion reserve in patients with ischemic heart disease. J Nucl Med. 2009;50:214–9. https://doi.org/10.2967/jnumed.108.054395.

16. Schenker MP, Dorbala S, Hong EC, et al. Interrelation of coronary calcification, myocardial ischemia, and outcomes in patients with intermediate likelihood of coronary artery disease: a combined positron emission tomography/computed tomography study. Circulation. 2008;117:1693–700. https://doi.org/10.1161/CIRCULATIONAHA.107.717512.
17. Lee SE, Nguyen C, Xie Y, et al. Recent advances in cardiac magnetic resonance imaging. Korean Circ J. 2019;49(2):146–59. https://doi.org/10.4070/kcj.2018.0246.
18. Haaf P, Garg P, Messroghli DR, et al. Cardiac T1 mapping and extracellular volume (ECV) in clinical practice: a comprehensive review. J Cardiovasc Magn Reason. 2016;18:89.
19. Sado DM, Flett AS, Banypersad SM, et al. Cardiovascular magnetic resonance measurement of myocardial extracellular volume in health and disease. Heart. 2012;98:1436–41. https://doi.org/10.1136/heartjnl-2012-302346.
20. Hinojar R, Varma N, Child N, et al. T1 mapping in discrimination of hypertrophic phenotypes: hypertensive heart disease and hypertrophic cardiomyopathy: findings from the international T1 multicenter cardiovascular magnetic resonance study. Circ Cardiovasc Imaging. 2015;8:8.
21. Puntmann VO, Voigt T, Chen Z, et al. Native T1 mapping in differentiation of normal myocardium from diffuse disease in hypertrophic and dilated cardiomyopathy. JACC Cardiovasc Imaging. 2013;6:475–84. https://doi.org/10.1016/j.jcmg.2012.08.019.
22. Verbrugge FH, Bertrand PB, Willems E, et al. Global myocardial oedema in advanced decompensated heart failure. Eur Heart J Cardiovasc Imaging. 2017;18:787–94. https://doi.org/10.1093/ehjci/jew131.
23. Bohnen S, Radunski UK, Lund GK, et al. Performance of T1 and T2 mapping cardiovascular magnetic resonance to detect active myocarditis in patients with recent-onset heart failure. Circ Cardiovasc Imaging. 2015;8:8.
24. McCrohon JA, Moon JC, Prasad SK, et al. Differentiation of heart failure related to dilated cardiomyopathy and coronary artery disease using gadolinium-enhanced cardiovascular magnetic resonance. Circulation. 2003;108:54–9. https://doi.org/10.1161/01.CIR.0000078641.19365.4C.
25. Kim RJ, Wu E, Rafael A, et al. The use of contrast-enhanced magnetic resonance imaging to identify reversible myocardial dysfunction. N Engl J Med. 2000;343:1445–53. https://doi.org/10.1056/NEJM200011163432003.
26. Dzeja PP, Redfield MM, Burnett JC, Terzic A. Failing energetics in failing hearts. Curr Cardiol Rep. 2000;2:212–7. https://doi.org/10.1007/s11886-000-0071-9.
27. Hundley WG, Bluemke DA, Finn JP, et al. ACCF/ACR/AHA/NASCI/SCMR 2010 expert consensus document on cardiovascular magnetic resonance: a report of the American College of Cardiology Foundation task force on expert consensus documents. J Am Coll Cardiol. 2010;55:2614–62.
28. Mukherjee R, Sprouse C, Pinheiro A, et al. Computing myocardial motion in 4D echocardiography. Ultrasound Med Biol. 2012;38(7):1284–97. https://doi.org/10.1016/j.ultrasmedbio.2012.03.007.
29. Hernandez-Suarez DF, Lopez-Candales A. Strain imaging echocardiography: what imaging cardiologists should know. Curr Cardiol Rev. 2017;13(2):118–29. https://doi.org/10.2174/1573403X12666161028122649.
30. Mirsky I, Parmley WW. Assessment of passive elastic stiffness for isolated heart muscle and the intact heart. Circ Res. 1973;33:233–43. https://doi.org/10.1161/01.RES.33.2.233.
31. Leung DY, Edin F, Ng AC. Emerging clinical role of strain imaging in echocardiography. Heart Lung Circ. 2010;19:161–74. https://doi.org/10.1016/j.hlc.2009.11.006.
32. Meyer MC, Mooney RP, Sekera AK. A critical pathway for patients with acute chest pain and low risk for short-term adverse cardiac events: role of outpatient stress testing. Ann Emerg Med. 2006;47(5):427–35. https://doi.org/10.1016/j.annemergmed.2005.10.010.
33. Scheuermeyer F, Innes G, Grafstein E, et al. Safety and efficiency of a chest pain diagnostic algorithm with selective outpatient stress testing for emergency department patients with potential ischemic chest pain. Ann Emerg Med. 2012;59(4):256–64. https://doi.org/10.1016/j.annemergmed.2011.10.016.

34. Cotarlan V, Ho D, Pineda J, Qureshi A, Shirani J. Impact of clinical predictors and routine coronary artery disease testing on outcome of patients admitted to chest pain decision unit. Clin Cardiol. 2014;37(3):146–51. https://doi.org/10.1002/clc.22229.
35. Kaufmann PA, Camici PG. Myocardial blood flow measurement by PET: technical aspects and clinical applications. J Nucl Med. 2005;46:75–88.
36. Jiang W, Chalich Y, Deen MJ. Sensors for positron emission tomography applications. Sensors. 2019;19(5019):1–56.

Atrial Fibrillation

5

Eric E. Harrison

Having to change the textbook is a big challenge.

—Dr. Charalambos Antoniades, Cardiology.

Abstract

When I used to walk through the hospital at night, I would find three elderly ladies with atrial fibrillation and a stroke. Thirty years later, a lot has changed and these are prevented! Many orthopedic medical centers have elective patients come in from out of town for TJA on the day of arrival. They have not been evaluated by the cardiologists. The cardiologists function as an emergency response team: they are called if there is an emergency much like fire rescue. Patients are not pre-evaluated.

Our patients are mostly regional so they are seen about a month before surgery by the orthopedists for TJA and referred to us if over 65 years of age or have a cardiac history. We take a day's visit to do the ultrasounds, echocardiogram with speckle tracking stain imaging, and CCTA (used in our OSCARS anatomical assessment—Orthopaedic Surgery Cardiovascular Assessment Risk Score) and evaluate the new patient. If we need more information, we will send them home with a heart rate and rhythm monitor (e.g., ZIO, Bardy), or a 24-h BP recorder, or both! They may start therapy, such as enhanced BP treatment, if there is inadequate BP control or they can return for further discussion and

E. E. Harrison (✉)
Board Chair International Cardio-Oncology Society, ICOS CEO PrivaCors Inc. Cardio-Orthopaedics®, Tampa, FL, USA

Morsani College of Medicine, Tampa, FL, USA

Joint Special Operations University, MacDill Air Force Base, Tampa, FL, USA

E. E. Harrison, N. H. Ho (eds.), *Managing Cardiovascular Risk In Elective Total Joint Arthroplasty*, https://doi.org/10.1007/978-3-031-26415-3_5

treatment. The point is that we've got a month to get them on the right pathway before surgery based on the anatomical data we have accumulated rapidly and not based on their exercise history which may have been nonexistent for months to years. This is the most reliable study of the preoperative anatomical findings of elective TJA patients and changes in treatment course 30 days before surgery with postoperative 90-day course in bundled patients. We did compare the patients to non-study and treatment group patients in other bundled groups that were not study patients who were cleared for surgery in the traditional method and operated on by these orthopedists in the group at various times when our bundled groups matched with cohorts. This data is available in presentations to ISTA by Dr. Kenneth Gustke (see reference). Without this interrupted information from the bundling changes, this is still an observational study and therefore falls short of a randomized study. Whether now after these observations of cardiovascular disease complications that can be treated and prevented, a randomized study may not be feasible, so this study provides detailed anatomical data on an observational level.

Keywords

Total Hip Arthroplasty (THA) · Total Knee Arthroplasty (TKA) · Atrial Fibrillation (AF) · Paroxysmal Atrial Fibrillation (PAF) · ZIO · Orthopaedic Surgery Cardiovascular Assessment Risk Score (OSCARS) · Chronic Atrial Fibrillation (CAF) · Left Ventricular Hypertrophy (LVH) · Pre-Ventricular Contractions (PVC) · Deep Venous Thrombosis (DVT)

5.1 Case 1 Presentation: Simple Case

Patient is a 78-year-old white female who is being evaluated for right THA in 30 days. She has been found on echocardiogram to have left ventricular hypertrophy of 14 mm and 15 mm of the in septum and inferior wall, respectively. She has no history of hypertension, but BP is 143/85 and 155/100. She has no history of diabetes. Her echocardiogram shows ejection fraction of 60% and LVH. Patient's carotid shows minimal carotid disease. She had a history of occasional palpitations, she said, basically once in a while. She has known hypothyroidism treated with the proper dose of deleted l-thyroxine 132 μg. With thyroid control with normal TSH, GERD, DVT, but a history of depression. Her CIMT showed minimal carotid disease. Her EKG showed right bundle branch block, normal sinus rhythm, left anterior fascicular block, and PVCS. She had a recording of her heartbeat by ZIO because of left ventricular hypertrophy and occasional palpitations. This revealed that she had undiagnosed paroxysmal atrial fibrillation very frequently although she had only occasional symptoms of palpitations. She had no history of sleep apnea which is also a cause of atrial fibrillation. It was felt that her left ventricular hypertrophy was an undiagnosed disease, i.e., hypertension which with female sex and age × 2, PAF would give her a CHADSVASC reading of four including newly diagnosed and untreated hypertension.

This patient has minimal coronary calcific remodeled nodules but LVH with undiagnosed hypertension and paroxysmal atrial fibrillation confirmed by ZIO.

This was time to start her on treatment for hypertension with the antihypertensive azilsartan medoxomil 80 mg with chlorthalidone 12.5 mg QD and nebivolol 10 mg qd and to continue this medication even on the day of surgery without interruption by taking the pill with sips of water. The patient will also be started on a DOAC, apixaban 5 mg bid, hold for 48 h before surgery and resume after surgery.

Patient will be put on antiarrhythmic medications which are dronedarone 400 mg bid and ranolazine 500 mg bid (off label use). Start now and continue even to the day of surgery without interruption, taking on the day of surgery with sips of water in the morning and 12 h later in the afternoon. These are two BID medications. Patient was seen two more times in follow-up prior to her TJA. There was no anesthesia preference. By this treatment regimen: the patient did not have a stroke, did not have paroxysmal atrial fibrillation and was not readmitted to the hospital. She could have had her THA surgery in an outpatient facility.

5.2 Case 2 Presentation: More Complex Case

This patient is a 73-year-old white female from Germany who is scheduled to have right TKA . She has a history of hypertension and is taking atenolol 50 mg daily. She also has a sinus bradycardia on her EKG because of the atenolol. Her echocardiogram showed she had mild to moderate aortic regurgitation, normal ejection fraction, and left ventricular hypertrophy of 13 and 14 septum and posterior wall, respectively. She had a Zio which showed paroxysmal atrial fibrillation. She had a history of having some atypical cerebral symptoms and had a brain MRI that showed multiple strokes. This is an example of recurrent CVAs. Our plan was to treat her with different medications since the atenolol she is on for hypertension is causing a sinus bradycardia. Her atenolol was stopped and she was started on azilsartan medoxomil 80 mg daily and chlorthalidone 25 mg a day as well as KCL 10 milliequivalents daily. She was also started on antiarrhythmics including dronedarone 400 mg bid and ranolazine 500 mg bid. She was started on a DOAC as well, which was apixaban 5 mg bid.

The patient cancelled her TKA and scheduled back surgery which was completed without problems. She returned a year later and was found that she had stopped her dronedarone and ranolazine and was taking propafenone Sr 325 mg BID instead. She still had hypertension and LVH . Repeat Zio showed 8% breakthrough of paroxysmal atrial fibrillation ranging from 93 to 190, average 145, the longest lasting 4 h 27 min. Her resting EKG was normal. Echocardiogram again showed moderate aortic regurgitation, moderate LVH, and a normal ejection fraction. She had a coronary CTA which showed a CAD-RADs 1 which meant that she had minimal nonobstructive calcific plaques. Her CIMT showed minimal carotid plaque. She was rescheduled for right TKA. She was considered low risk for surgery with instructions to hold her Xarelto 48 h before the surgery but continue the dronedarone and ranolazine on the surgery day with sips of water and medications BID. Her right TKA was completed and she did well. She returned again for a left TKA and did well also.

5.3 Case Review: Not Reproduced

For most pre-op cases, a typical pre-op cardiac evaluation by a "binary"(to stent or not stent) cardiologist may overlook many of the patient's current problems and opt for approval to proceed with surgery based on ECG and Echo (Fig. 5.3). Below, I detail my experiences as I summarize the above two cases and drill deeper into exploring innovative ways to actually consider the patient's associated conditions more fully and move away from "binary" thinking.

These two cases summarize the findings in two patients with unrecognized and therefore untreated hypertension. I don't have an opportunity to record a lot of random blood pressures prior to the patient's appointment. So I might not make the diagnosis from one blood pressure alone in the clinic although if elevated that may be a clue to hypertension or it could be white coat syndrome. The EKG may be helpful by showing prominent voltage although that is not always present. Therefore, it was a good decision to check the required pre-op CCTA for LVH by measuring the LV thickness routinely as a clue. The other clue would be to have the echo technologist carefully measure the LV thickness at the level of the Chordae tendineae papillary muscle junction during diastole. They both had undiagnosed LVH which is a clue that they either have hypertension or sleep apnea, both lead to LVH. LVH leads to diastolic LV dysfunction and elevated left atrial (LA) pressure. This leads to LA expansion and enlargement which then leads to LA fibrosis which can be detected byLA MRI. We will reach the point that it is irreversible unless we intervene. The LA expansion can be detected both by the CCTA in diastole and by the echocardiogram. This LA scar tissue is the set up for the generation of PACs and atrial fibrillation or flutter [1].

I was one of the 18 cardiac MRI experts participating in DECAAF 1, along with 18 cardiac EP doctors who were referenced in the landmark JAMA published paper. DECAAF processors would grade atrial fibrosis by sophisticated MRI contrast colored pattern recognition and be able to classify and correlate the amount of fibrotic LA tissue with the ability to recognize the presence of atrial fibrillation not dependent on the amount of fibrosis but also recognize the ability to ablate the AF, this time because of the amount and distribution of fibrosis (Fig. 5.1).

It is useful in predicting atrial fibrillation in those who would get it in the future. Dr. Alexis Harrison demonstrated normal MRIs in a cohort of patients getting colonoscopy [2]. Dr. Paul Bansmann, MD in Cologne demonstrated that MRI is a good screen for predicting the onset of AF if the LA is enlarged and that the LA fibrosis

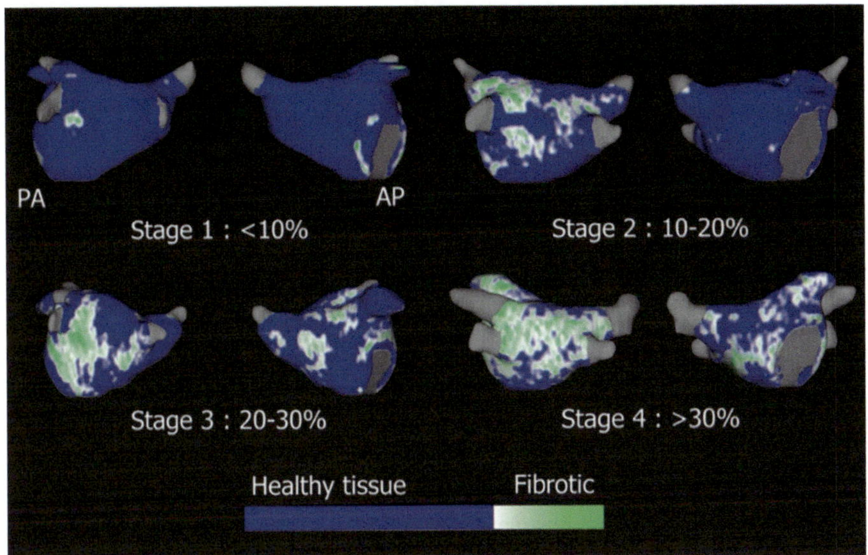

Fig. 5.1 Sophisticated MRI contrast colored pattern recognition

exceeds that of normal shown by Dr. A. Harrison. I had thought about using DECAAF-derived LA MRI with gadolinium contrast in these patients to recognize the presence of LA fibrosis as a sign that the patient may have AF but realized that it would take too long and would increase the expense.

After the discovery of occult undiagnosed LVH and hypertension or sleep apnea with possibly some LA enlargement, the next step was to put the patients on a monitoring device like the ZIO for 3 days to a week, depending on the time available, to find atrial fibrillation/flutter to know that the patient has this and to time the duration to decide if it was significant. Other options if time was not a problem would be the use of KardiaMobile 6 L by Dr. David Albert or another AliveCor device, a smartphone such as iPhone or Garmin to find A "Smartwatch Algorithm for Automated Detection of Atrial Fibrillation" [3].

On the other hand, cardiologists have been exposed recently to challenges in the screening for asymptomatic AF with Smartwatches, Fitness trackers, and other wearable EKG recorders. There is not enough data to explore the pros and cons of this data.

If we are unsure about the hypertension, we do a 24-h BP recording which takes a BP with a cuff hourly whether he/she is awake or asleep. Also if bp is normal we can send them a sleep study device for overnight recording looking for sleep apnea and pulse oximetry drops during sleep. A third possibility would be hypertrophic cardiomyopathy or other cardiomyopathies which can be another cause of AF.

Here are a list of findings that make it a bit easier to predict PAF: FH + for AF, PACs, LVH, LAE, history of AF, 3–7 day Zio, palpitations, CABG with postoperative AF and AF years later, pericarditis, (DECAF), Ibrutinib, abnormal EKG, genetic testing of a 32-gene screening test. Patients in the highest tercile had a 31% rate of ischemic stroke in mean follow-up of 2.8 years compared to the lowest tercile and 3.5 greater risk of stroke but with a CHA2DS2-VASc of 1–2.

Our patients in chronic atrial fibrillation were not good candidates for evaluating their coronaries by CCTA because of their irregular heart rate and our CT equipment. We could do calcium scoring but that had artifact. This group on medical therapy with anticoagulation medications and drugs for rate control seemed less likely to have a risk of CVA with intermittent interruption of their anticoagulation for TJA. Further studies will be useful.

However, PAF occurred irregularly and infrequently that the heart was regular most of the time. We have used beta blockers for heart rate control in NSR when the rate is above 60. We just had to slow it down with a betablocker. Recently, we switched to Ivabradine as an effective heart rate lowering treatment given an hour before surgery. This can induce atrial fibrillation and needs to be avoided in those with underlying PAF. This is another reason to be aware that your patient has PAF which reduces symptoms in chronic stable angina and reduces hospitalizations in chronic heart failure. Ivabradine may carry an increased risk of atrial fibrillation.

We graded the lesions coronary stenosis lesions by a CCTA score published in SCCT. CAD-RADs Scores were 0 (7), 1 (8), 2 (7), 3 (2), 4 (1), 5 (1), some with a past history of normal caths [4] and one calcium score only of a patient with chronic AF of 17. Thus in this group, paroxysmal atrial fibrillation was rarely caused by significant CAD or previous CABG!

Paroxysmal Atrial Fibrillation is predictable in patients with HTN and even more so with LVH. The echo gives the best evidence of HTN being borderline at 12 mm and enlarged beyond that measurement. Left atrial enlargement is key if above 5 cm on the 2D or 3D modes. Severe mitral regurgitation is another hint. Frequent PACs is also a predictor. Giving a family history of AF or giving a personal history of palpitations is suggestive.

Recording the Zio is the most reliable predictor of PAF, the longer recording, the most reliable yield. If we have a week to record, that is very helpful, but sometimes the clearance is rushed and we only have 3 days.

We reviewed an earlier patient population and found that 72% of our TJA group had HTN, 74 with known HTN and 10 more with undiagnosed HTN with LVH and elevated BP requiring treatment preoperatively. Of the patients with HTN, 59% had LVH.

Why is atrial fibrillation and flutter so important in cardio-orthopedics as to deserve a whole chapter and to devise a way to discover it in our group of pre-op patients over 65 for elective TJA? Elizabeth Bernstein wrote a unique article in the Personal Column of the WSJ entitled "After a Lifetime of Sailing Together, My dad Assed Me for One Last Favor" right before Father's Day. Her father was a Miami orthopedist who needed hip replacement. The night of the operation, he had a massive stroke with aphasia, inability to understand language. He survived like that for 3years(https://www.wsj.com/articles/fathers-day-after-a-lifetime-of-sailing-together-my-dad-asked-me-for-one-last-favor-11655155439).

From causing an irregular heartbeat with a rapid rate accompanied by sometimes symptomatic palpitations and sometimes hypotension to causing a CVA/TIA if persisting too long (sometimes greater than 24 h). The treatment involves the use of drugs for rate control, other drugs as antiarrhythmics, and the addition of anticoagulants to prevent strokes but which can promote bleeding from a new surgical site. Thus, you can see avoidance of the anticoagulant by the recommended guidelines can be the safest course if possible prior to TJA.

On the other hand, those who had carotid testing were at no risk of CVA/TIA in our group for elective TJA, all who had no or minimal carotid vascular disease. I had always thought that the cause of CVA/TIA in these patients was severe carotid vascular disease, but this was nonexistent on the ultrasound of the carotids of all our patients! Specifically, what we were looking for was high grade carotid stenosis as seen in this picture.

Other possible threats were carotid plaque with lipid lake which could potentially rupture and accumulate platelets that could embolize or thrombose as well as a small plaque ulcer (Fig. 5.2). These were not present in our TJA group.

Another example that was not seen in our TJA group but was in a patient that had a TIA of uncertain cause, can be seen in (Fig. 5.3). Not reproduced.

How prevalent is AF in our elderly patient group? In 25% of the global population and growing, an epidemic of aging and in TJA of the lower extremity, a relative common complication. In patients over 60 with hypertension, the risk of AF increases in woman by 40% and in males by 50% [5].

For total hip or knee replacement, rheumatoid arthritis patients have a 605 greater risk of developing AF than those without. The Journal of Bone and Joint Surgery in

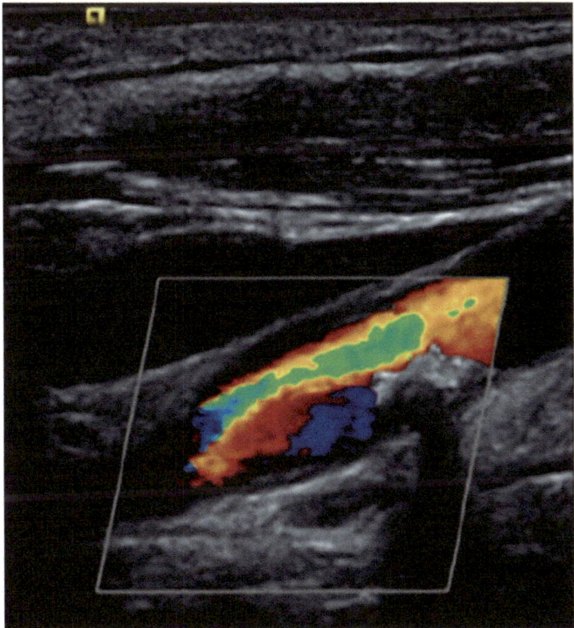

Fig. 5.2 LICA stenosis with a plaque that narrows the lumen which shows the color-coded increase in the velocity of flow. Not reproduced

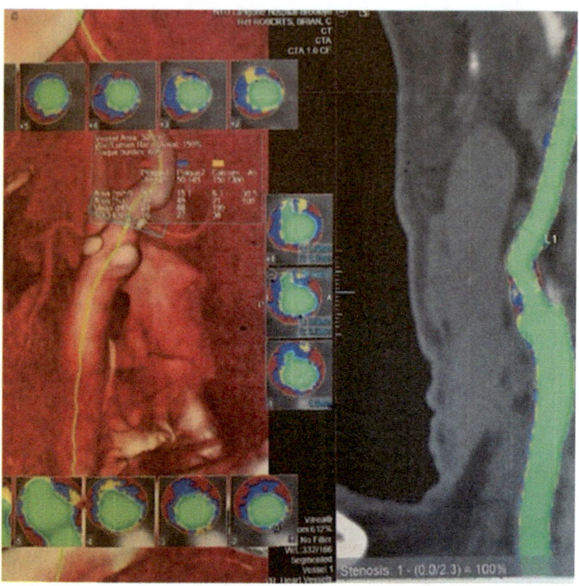

Fig. 5.3 Shows the LICA plaque with a lipid lake seen in red adjacent to the lumen in green with a small plaque ulcer seen as a 1.8 by 2.0 mm outpouching of the green lumen cross-sectional area. The area of lumen stenosis was only 18%. MASKED?

2013 reported that patients reported in smaller patient groups such as 131 patients in Poland with age of 69, 5.9% had AF. I'm unsure as to whether they were monitored and how long [4].

The prevalence of atrial fibrillation in our group of 430 patients over 65 years old for elective TJA was 68 or 15.8%. Of these patients, 38 (56%) had PAF with the other 30 (44%) having chronic AF. PAF patients are just as likely as chronic AF patients to get CVAs/TIAs. In actuality, I suspect that those with PAF are more likely to get embolic episodes in my experience since they are going in and out of AF which is a risk factor. As an aside, the incidence of atrial fibrillation over the age of 65 years old in acute elderly patient was 28.1% that is 247 out of 861 suggesting atrial fibrillation is more common in this population [6]. These patients also were found to have longer stay length of stay [7, 8].

We have a lot of information about this group of patients for elective TJA when they are compared to another group of patients from the CABANA Trial (Fig. 5.4) [9] which I participated in and enrolled patients. This study was catheter ablation of atrial fibrillation versus drug therapy results. In this group of patients, 44% were PAF. CABANA was a younger group with 66% males and 64% females were over 65 years old were as our patients were 89% over 65 years old. Community trial was an international study of 140 center clinical trials patients designated to randomized 2200 patients to a strategy of catheter ablation versus state-of-the-art rate or rhythm control drug therapy.

The risk factors in the CABANA trial group of patients fit the risk of cardiac-orthopedic patients quite nicely. Criteria that they used were over the age of 65 or less than 65 years old with one or more risk factors for stroke: hypertension, diabetes, congestive heart failure or prior stroke. Other risk factors were atherosclerotic

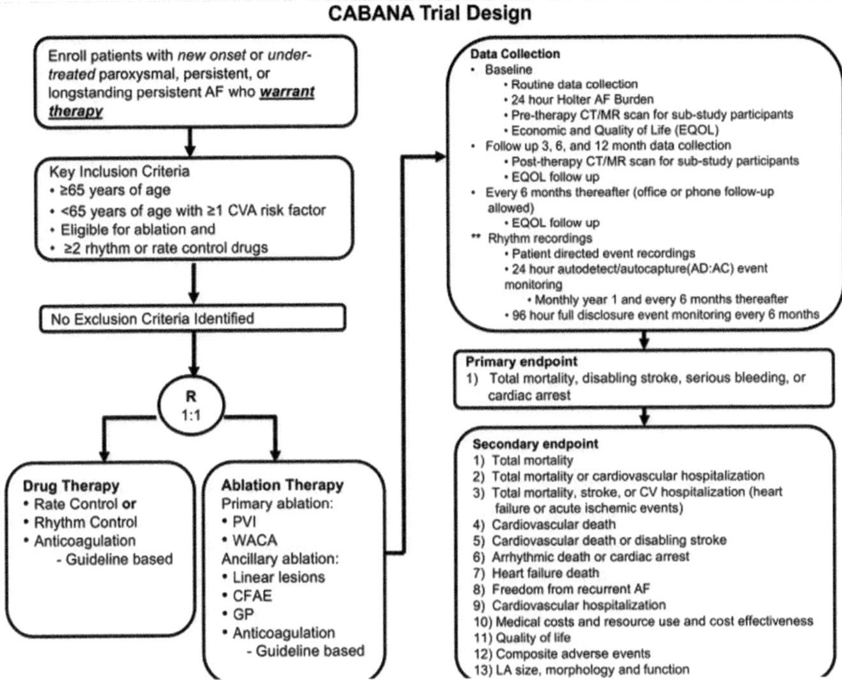

Fig. 5.4 CABANA trial design (Packer DL, Mark DB, et al. Catheter Ablation versus Antiarrhythmic Drug Therapy for Atrial Fibrillation (CABANA) Trial: Study Rationale and Design. Am Heart J. 2018 May;199:192–199)

vascular disease, left atrial size greater than 5.0 cm, or ejection fraction less than or equal to 35%, patients less than 65 years of age and the only risk factor of hypertension must have a second risk factor or LV hypertrophy to qualify.

In the CABANA Trial conclusion, ablation did not produce a significant reduction in the primary endpoint and all-cause mortality. The primary outcome death disabling stroke serious bleeding or cardiac arrest at 5 years for ablation versus drug therapy was 8% versus 9.2%.

Because of our patients being similar to those in CABANA and the outcome of ablation versus drug therapy being the same, we did not consider RFA in our patients either as the first time or repeat ablation if they had broken through but considered anticoagulation with DOACs and antiarrhythmic drugs or rate control.

If we are going to accept our role of controlling the arrythmia with antiarrhythmic medications or rate control and anticoagulation, I am going to fixate on PAF since I believe this offers the greatest risk in the short period of time of anticoagulation suspension perioperatively. We follow the rules of suspending the DOAC according to written guidelines. This period of time seems to be better tolerated in chronic AF as opposed to an increased risk with PAF going in and out of the arrythmia and having a greater risk of thrombosis at this time. Unfortunately, we do not have proof of this hypothesis. What we do have is an opportunity for elective TJA patients to have their PAF discontinued with AF drugs which can be continued perioperatively including the taking of the medications with sips of water on the day of surgery during the time of suspension of DOACs and compare these patients who don't have this done with PAF (a Cohort) and also compare these groups with patients with chronic AF with a period of DOAC suspension to avoid bleeding complications with TJA.

Unfortunately, the data we need is not available. A couple of points of interest from a recent article suggests [10]: Firstly, "The strongest evidence suggests that patients with persistent AF are at higher risk of stroke than those with paroxysmal AF; however, the relationship of increasing AF burden with risk of stroke is not well characterized. CIED-based studies conclude that higher AF burden is associated with higher risk of stroke, but it is unclear whether the risk increases continuously or whether a threshold exists, in large part because of variable AF duration cutoffs, which were mostly arbitrarily prespecified rather than empirically derived. The effect of very brief AF episodes of <5–6 min on stroke risk has not been rigorously evaluated and remains unknown." Secondly, they also state that "Remaining knowledge gaps indicate the need for future studies, including those focused on validation of definitions and measures of AF burden, determination of the threshold of AF burden that results in an increased risk of stroke that warrants anticoagulation, and discovery of the mechanisms underlying the weak temporal correlations of AF and stroke."

This data does not state what I need to know about PAF versus CAF stroke risk during a short time of anticoagulation absence. The Bridge theory with stopping a DOAC and substituting IV lovenox has been denied as a useful option. "For most patients, we do not use bridging anticoagulation (use of a short-acting parenteral agent to reduce the interval without anticoagulation), because it increases bleeding risk without reducing the rate of thromboembolism. However, some patients on warfarin with an especially high thromboembolic risk (e.g., mechanical heart valve, recent stroke) may benefit from bridging (see 'Bridging anticoagulation' below.)" Thus, I only bridge those with prosthetic mechanical valves.

If we are going to stop the DOAC and not bridge, then we need to continue the anticoagulant the patient is on with sips of water on the morning of surgery. Therefore, a working knowledge of the classes of drugs, other drug interactions, half-lives, electrolyte management, complications with CAD and LV dysfunction, management with renal or liver dysfunction CHA2DS2VASv score, HAS-BLED score and other factors need to be taken into consideration. These scores may be summarized.

The two main guidance criteria for AF continue to be HAS-BLED (Hypertension, abnormal renal/liver function, stroke, bleeding history. Labile INR, elderly, drugs) and CHA2DS2-VASc (Congestive heart failure, hypertension, age, diabetes, previous stroke/TIA,—vascular disease).

Fortunately, when dealing with the classes and drugs for preventing AF, I have had the experience of running experiment research studies on all the drugs with FDA-issued INDS and in cooperation with all the major world-wide drug companies over the years with research involving bretylium tosylate, amiodarone, dronedarone, flecainide, lidocaine, dofetilide, mexiletine, procainamide, Quinidine, potassium, ibutilide, ivabradine, and others. I would not want to review the strengths and weakness of each medication and combinations but would like to simply state want we did with our study patients and the results of their treatment.

The combination of dronedarone (multaq) and ranolazine has been extremely useful in preventing atrial fibrillation (Fig. 5.5). We have not had a single break through case in this group. We had one patient that PAF was prevented in the hospital but who broke through after 1 week after discharge who was converted by increasing the ranolazine to 1000 mg bid.

An 82-year-old male with PAF who is going to have a surgical procedure and is sent for patient clearance. Instructions are sent to the referring physician for discontinuing Eliquis 5 mg bid 48 h before surgery and continuing daily including multaq 400 mg bid and ranaxa 500 mg bid the day of surgery with sips of water. Unfortunately, the patient was instructed by the surgery team to discontinue all medications 1 week before surgery and never received my personal instructions. He showed up on his procedure day in PAF with a mild stroke.

From here on out we would give the patient himself my special instructions and the patient will take the responsibility even to the point of carrying and administering the antiarrhythmic drugs himself.

The following slide shows the medications that everyone took the day of surgery. They stayed on the drug they were taking including on the operative day by taking the pill with sips of water in the early AM prior to surgery. Those that had successful ablation were on no medications if we proved the absence of PAF. Likewise, the patient who had his LA appendage successfully closed with the Watchman had no medications. Those who were not on antiarrhythmic medications were given ranolazine 500 mg bid plus dronedarone 80 mg bid.

None of the PAF patients developed PAF perioperatively (Fig. 5.6). One patient had a Watchman procedure with the placement of an occluding device over the atrial appendage which prevents emboli. Ninety percent of clots from the heart form in the atrial appendage which leads to strokes.

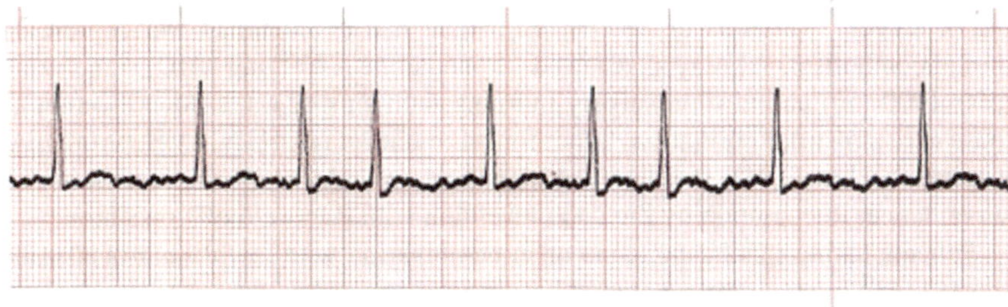

Fig. 5.5 EKG strip of atrial fibrillation and prevention by ranolazine and dronedarone. Not reproduced

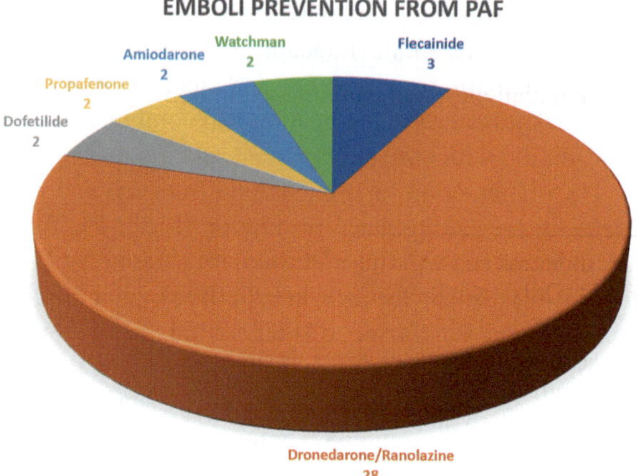

Fig. 5.6 the therapy for preventing atrial fibrillation in the TJA patients with PAF. Not reproduced

The Harmony study showed that patients with PAF treated with dronedarone and ranolazine in appropriate but lower doses than clinically available in the USA had a 59% rate of not developing AF in a year. This is better than the results from the use of amiodarone [11].

We had our own experience with a group of patients with PAF who were treated with dronedarone and ranolazine who were not TJA candidates: Frequently, they had failed Propafenone. These were not TJA patients but had various medical problems and PAF. Eighteen patients had suppression of PAF and did well on the combination drugs. Two were successfully treated with ranolazine alone. Of the AF group of TJA patients, 68 patients had AF, 38 PAF. Patient anatomy and treatment: 2 with significant mitral valve disease, 1 gross tricuspid abnormality, 1 resolved cardiomyopathy, 1 severe CAD. CAD-RADs Scores: 0 (7 patients), 1 (8), 2 (7), 3 (2), 4 (1), 5 (1). Seven normal catheterizations, and 1 chronic AF with calcium score of 17.2 had multiple CVAs, 1 a single CVA, 3 sleep apnea. 1 RFA ×3 continued PAF and a later TIA. Two with RFA ×1 continued PAF, and 2 others RFA did not have AF (Fig. 5.7). Fifteen with PAF took no anti-coagulation medication; 23 were on anticoagulants. Many had unknown HTN and LVH. Of PAF patients, 2 were treated with dofetilide, 3 flecainide, 2 propafenone, and 2 amiodarone including the morning of surgery with sips of water. One patient had a watchman which prevents thromboembolism. The rest received dronedarone (400 mg BID) ranolazine (500–1000 mg) and also on surgery morning with sips of water. Identification of those at risk of atrial fibrillation /flutter for surveillance, i.e., HTN, LVH, prior RFA, palpitations, hx of SVT. Pre-bundling Identification of Atrial Fibrillation/Flutter by surveillance: Recognition by Zio and prevention with Ranolazine/Dronedarone.

Patients taking ranolazine alone or in combination with low-dose dronedarone showed QTc interval prolongation. Our observations of low-dose ranolazine alone for patients who cannot tolerate combinations with dronedarone reveals that very few respond as an antiarrhythmic, but those that do respond can take it indefinitely. We used readily available dosages (standard dosing recommended by manufacturer). Ranolazine is currently approved as an antianginal agent in patients with

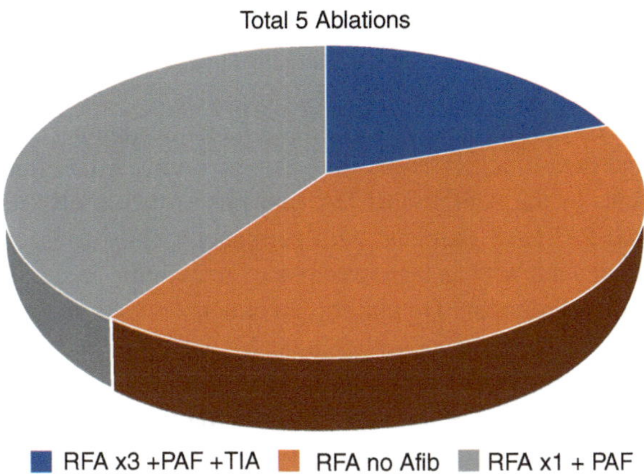

Fig. 5.7 This group of patients were the group that had ablation. Not reproduced

chronic angina (class IIA). Ranolazine's antiarrhythmic effects are due to predominant inhibition of late sodium current and the rapid potassium rectifier current as well as late ICa and INa-Ca. It also suppresses the early and delayed after depolarizations. These may be promising new treatment options for AF, especially in patients with HF, and warrant further clinical investigation. Several studies demonstrated no significant complications from the use of these drugs in combination [12]. The development of a promising drug, namely, Gilead's fixed-dose combination of ranolazine/dronedarone: P16 Mar 2017 Discontinued—Phase II for PAF in the USA, the UK, Poland, Netherlands, Italy, Israel, and Germany (PO) because dronedarone/ranolazine was not listed on Gilead pipeline of March 2017. On 10 May 2014, final efficacy data from the phase II HARMONY trial in PAF released by Gilead Sciences. Then finally, on 31 Mar 2014 Gilead Sciences completes the phase II HARMONY trial in PAF in the USA, Germany, Israel, Italy, Netherlands, Poland, and the UK (NCT01522651).

It is important to realize that combining these two drugs that affect the QT interval can result in significant arrhythmias in certain patients with rare congenital long QT syndrome or other cardiac diseases (e.g., sarcoid, amyloid, Fabry's, TOF repair) [13]. Low doses of ranolazine and dronedarone in combination exert potent protection against atrial fibrillation and vulnerability to ventricular arrhythmias during acute MI [14]. Conclusions from Verrier, et al.: Combined administration of low doses of ranolazine and dronedarone exerts a potent antiarrhythmic action on ischemia-induced vulnerability to AF and ventricular tachyarrhythmias due to direct effects on myocardial electrical properties.

It is important to note there are several reported drug–drug interactions. A careful audit of the drugs' manufacturer labels is paramount to make sure patients are well taken care of. Do not take ranolazine if you take any of the following medicines for fungus infection (ketoconazole, itraconazole), for bacterial infection (clarithromycin), for depression (nefazodone), for HIV (nelfinavir, ritonavir, lopinavir and ritonavir, indinavir, saquinavir), for tuberculosis (rifampin, rifabutin, rifapentine), for seizures (phenobarbital, phenytoin, carbamazepine), and the herbal supplement St. John's wort.

Drug–drug Interactions with dronedarone include: Treatment with Class I or III antiarrhythmics or drugs that are strong inhibitors of CYP 3A must be stopped before starting MULTAQ, patients should be instructed to avoid grapefruit juice beverages while taking MULTAQ. Calcium channel blockers with depressant effects and beta-blockers could increase the bradycardia effects of MULTAQ on conduction. In the ANDROMEDA (patients with recently decompensated heart failure) and PALLAS (patients with permanent AFib) trials, baseline use of digoxin was associated with an increased risk of arrhythmic or sudden death in MULTAQ-treated patients compared to placebo. In patients not taking digoxin, no difference in risk of sudden death was observed in the MULTAQ vs placebo groups Digoxin can potentiate the electrophysiologic effects of MULTAQ (such as decreased AV-node conduction). MULTAQ increases exposure to digoxin. Consider discontinuing digoxin. If digoxin treatment is continued, halve the dose of digoxin, monitor serum levels closely, and observe for toxicity. Postmarketing cases of increased INR with or without bleeding events have been reported in warfarin-treated patients initiated with MULTAQ. Monitor INR after initiating MULTAQ in patients taking warfarin. Avoid simvastatin doses greater than 10 mg daily. Follow statin label recommendations for use with CYP 3A and P-gP inhibitors such as MULTAQ.

Our research shows a small sample of 26 patients that had PAF done with coronary CTA demonstrated their cardiac anatomy, of which three had cautions (yellow arrows) and one had an MI that was predicted by our Sherlock Analysis successfully treated post-MI resulting in no cardiac damage. Patients who develop AF after TJA in the hospital may not be good candidates for electrical cardioversion because of the sudden muscle contraction from the electrical shock. This may damage the new prosthetic device. Using ibutilide for cardioversion pharmacologically within 12 h of the onset of AF or TEE/ibutilide after 12 h but within 48 h is a reasonable approach to avoid the sudden jump of muscle contraction.

We have never had the opportunity to cardiovert a patient who newly went into AF in the hospital although we utilize the PAs for staffing the hospital and they did not report a cardioversion. We do have special guidelines that we will present that we developed for this regimen so that they would be converted by medical therapy without sedation and without the traumatic patient sudden jump and physical projection which could do damage to his/her new prosthetic knee or hip. We believe that a naïve patient of new AF could benefit from ibutilide therapy post-op because we don't want to electrically cardiovert them due to risk of dislodging the prosthesis. However, we would not recommend use of ibutilide on a patient who was concomitantly taking ranolazine and/or dronedarone. It is important to note that our patients who were on our regimen of dronedarone and ranolazine never went into AF perioperatively [15]. Rankin, et al. demonstrated in a subgroup analysis that even within 48 h, the risk of thromboembolism varied with the duration of AF, from 0.3% if the patient was cardioverted within 12 h compared with 1.1% beyond 12 h. Airaksinen et al. found that a delay to cardioversion of 12 h or longer from symptom onset was associated with greater risk of thromboembolic complications (1.1%) [16].

Nuoto et al. explains that stroke is the most serious complication of AF, and the risk of thromboembolic complications was 0.7% if cardioversion was done without anticoagulation within 48 h of onset of AF [17]. Even though studies do show that ibutilide appears to be an effective therapy for conversion of recent onset AFib and Aflutter in elderly patients, there is a risk for a rare complication of Torsades de pointes [18].

While we mainly treat with chemical conversion with ibutilide, if that fails, we will convert electrically, which has shown to have a 100% conversion rate of those patients who were pretreated with ibutilide as opposed to 72% with no pretreatment. Again, in this study, there was a 4% risk of Torsades de pointes and a 4.9% risk of monomorphic VTach, which will require close inpatient monitoring for at least 4 h postinfusion [19].

The following is a proposed protocol for ibutilide pretreatment for electrical cardioversion: (A) Class Ia antiarrhythmic drugs (Vaughan Williams Classification), such as disopyramide, quinidine, and procainamide, and other class III drugs, such as amiodarone and sotalol, should not be given concomitantly with Ibutilide Fumarate Injection or within 4 h postinfusion because of their potential to prolong refractoriness. In the clinical trials, class I or other class III antiarrhythmic agents were withheld for at least five half-lives prior to ibutilide infusion and for 4 h after dosing, but thereafter were allowed at the physician's discretion, (B) check Mg and K, EF >30%, (C) 1 mg ibutilide over 10 min. Observation period 10 min, (D) CV standard protocol, and finally, (D) there is up to a 4% risk of torsade de pointes and a 4.9% risk of monomorphic ventricular tachycardia. Hence, close monitoring in an intensive care unit setting is warranted during and at least for 4 h after drug infusion. The anticoagulation strategy is the same as for any other mode of cardioversion. If torsades, 2 g Mg sulfate (10 mL of a 20% solution) IV over 1 min. In 5 min if necessary, repeat, then follow by a 3–20 mg per min infusion [20, 21].

Patients in registration trials were hemodynamically stable. Patients with specific cardiovascular conditions such as symptomatic heart failure, recent acute myocardial infarction, and angina were excluded. About two thirds had cardiovascular symptoms, and the majority of patients had left atrial enlargement, decreased left ventricular ejection fraction, a history of valvular disease, or previous history of atrial fibrillation or flutter. Electrical cardioversion was allowed 90 min after the infusion was complete. Patients could be given other antiarrhythmic drugs 4 h postinfusion.

5.4 Conclusion

In our group of 430 patients who were evaluated anatomically by ultrasound and CCTA for TJA a month before cardiac clearance, 59% had PAF with 31% with persistent AF. Our group was 49% male and 51% female with 89% were over 65 years old. The age distribution was 5% in their 50 s, 6% 60–64 years of age, 7% 65–69, 47% in their 70 s, and 30% in their 80 s. Thirteen percent had AF although higher percentages were observed in of 28%. This group with AF is at high risk of stroke, complications and prolonged hospitalization. On the other hand, those who had carotid testing were at no risk of CVA/TIA in our group for elective TJA.

The risk factors in this Cabana group of patients fit the risks of Cardio-Orthopaedic patients quite nicely. Over the age of 65, and hypertension either diagnosed or undiagnosed along with accompanying LVH are very high risk in this assessment. Risk of a stroke by atherosclerotic vascular disease or LA size >5.0 cm is of interest as well. These are all parameters that we can observe with echo, carotid ultrasound, thoracic or abdominal ultrasound, and the thoracic aorta as viewed with CCTA, our anatomical assessment by OSCARs . The criteria of >2 drugs to be eligible exceeds the criteria of our undiagnosed patients with PAF which gives us greater opportunity with medications since the Cabana patients failed two drugs.

Our group of patients with PAF had complications leading to longer hospitalization in treatment groups while out group with careful drug suppression with a combination of dronedarone and ranolazine did not have AF perioperatively with no prolongation requiring prolonged hospitalization.

We also designed a regimen of cardioversion if someone would breakthrough with PAF resulting in the use of Ibutilide to avoid complex electrical cardioversion with the risk of the muscular contraction resulting in joint prothesis dislodgement but fortunately this was not necessary to implement.

As far as prevention of atrial fibrillation when their TJA is resolved, this will require greater consideration and thought. New cardiologists don't get involved in treating PAF or chronic AF because this requires a lot of experience, thought, and expertise. They don't have the experience from the clinics promoted by drug companies to evaluate new drugs for arrhythmia in the past. I had FDA IND numbers for all the drugs that were developed in the past and acquired a great deal of experience from my very large clinics prior to the development of AF ablation which now has become commonplace in every hospital which has an EP Lab. No new drugs are being developed. The cardiologists have to shorten visits to accumulate RVUs (billable hours) and would not have the time to read up on antiarrhythmic medications. Absent this experience, young cardiologists will routinely send the patient with AF to an EP doctor and may not elect or TJA rhythm control in the absence of protection with an anticoagulant.

EP doctors have become very plentiful because of training programs, hospital EP lab development, and insurance and Medicare high reimbursement. Although the Cabana Study showed no difference in outcome between the drug therapy group of patients and the ablation group who had failed two drugs, there was crossover and other factors subtracting from the conclusion. The EP group has issued their own consensus statement advocating ablation if patients are symptomatic. If multiple ablations fail in their selected patients, then drug therapy is started. Then there is always the option of AV nodal ablation and a pacer versus heart rate control with beta blockers or calcium channel blockers. The EP doctors will have problems adopting this simple plan in their busy schedule. This is one of the reasons we have considered creating cardio-orthopedics as a new subspecialty of cardiology not unlike cardio-oncology which has been very successful as a subsection for the 10 years since the founding in addressing heart problems associated with cancer treatment.

References

1. Marrouche NF, Wilber D, Hindricks G, et al. Association of atrial tissue fibrosis identified by delayed enhancement MRI and atrial fibrillation catheter ablation: the DECAAF study. JAMA. 2014;311(5):498–506. https://doi.org/10.1001/jama.2014.3.
2. McGann C, Akoum N, Patel A, et al. Atrial fibrillation ablation outcome is predicted by left atrial remodeling on MRI. Circ Arrhythm Electrophysiol. 2014;7(1):23–30. https://doi.org/10.1161/CIRCEP.113.000689. Epub 2013 Dec 20
3. Bumgarner JM, Tarakji KG, et al. Smartwatch algorithm for automated detection of atrial fibrillation. J Am Coll Cardiol. 2018;71(21):2381–8.
4. Legosz P, Kotkowski M, Platek AE, et al. Assessment of cardiovascular risk in patients undergoing total joint alloplasty: the CRASH-JOINT study. Kardiol Pol. 2017;75(3):213–20. https://doi.org/10.5603/KP.a2016.0162. Epub 2016 Nov 23
5. Kannel WB, Wolf PA, Benjamin EJ, Levey D. Prevalence, incidence, prognosis, and predisposing conditions for atrial fibrillation: population-based estimates. Am J Cardiol. 1998;82(7 Suppl 1):2N–9N.
6. Impact of Atrial Fibrillation and anticoagulation in Elderly Hip Fracture surgery patients KT, IS, JC, SS, and MK Pesented at the 14th Annual Perioperative Medicine Summit, Orlando, Florida on 02/14/2019.
7. Tabatabaee RM, Rasouli MR, et al. Coronary revascularization and adverse events in joint arthroplasty. J Surg Res. 2015;198(1):135–42. https://doi.org/10.1016/j.jss.2015.05.013. Epub 2015 May 14
8. Aggarwal VK, Tischler EH, et al. Patients with atrial fibrillation undergoing total joint arthroplasty increase hospital burden. J Bone Joint Surg Am. 2013;95(17):1606–11. https://doi.org/10.2106/JBJS.L.00882.
9. Packer DL, Mark DB, et al. Catheter ablation versus antiarrhythmic drug therapy for atrial fibrillation (CABANA) trial: study rationale and design. Am Heart J. 2018;199:192–9.
10. Chen LY, Chung MK, Allen LA, et al. Atrial fibrillation burden: moving beyond atrial fibrillation as a binary entity: a scientific statement from the American Heart Association. Circulation. 2018;137:e623–44.
11. Reiffel JA, Camm AJ, Belardinelli L, et al. The HARMONY trial: combined Ranolazine and Dronedarone in the Management of Paroxysmal Atrial Fibrillation: mechanistic and therapeutic synergism. Circ Arrhythm Electrophysiol. 2015;8:1048–56.
12. Hartmann N, Mason FE, et al. The combined effects of ranolazine and dronedarone on human atrial and ventricular electrophysiology. Mol Cell Cardiol. 2016;94:95–106. https://doi.org/10.1016/j.yjmcc.2016.03.012. Epub 2016 Apr 4
13. Frommeyer G, Kaiser D, et al. Effect of ranolazine on ventricular repolarization in class III antiarrhythmic drug treated rabbits. Heart Rhythm. 2012;9(12):2051–8. https://doi.org/10.1016/j.hrthm.2012.08.029. Epub 2012 Aug 28
14. Verrier RL, et al. Low doses of ranolazine and dronedarone in combination exert potent protection against atrial fibrillation and vulnerability to ventricular arrhythmias during acute myocardial ischemia. Heart Rhythm. 2013;10(1):121–7.
15. Rankin AJ, Rankin SH. Cardioverting acute atrial fibrillation and the risk of thromboembolism: not all patients are created equal. Clin Med (Lond). 2017;17(5):419–23. https://doi.org/10.7861/clinmedicine.17-5-419.
16. Airaksinen KEJ, Grönberg T, Nuotio I, Nikkinen M, et al. Thromboembolic complications after cardioversion of acute atrial fibrillation: the FinCV (Finnish CardioVersion) study. J Am Coll Cardiol. 2013;62(13):1187–92. https://doi.org/10.1016/j.jacc.2013.04.089.
17. Nuotio I, Hartikainen JEK, et al. Time to cardioversion for acute atrial fibrillation and thromboembolic complications. JAMA. 2014;312(6):647–9. https://doi.org/10.1001/jama.2014.3824.

18. Gowda RM, Khan IA, Punukollu G, et al. Use of ibutilide for cardioversion of recent-onset atrial fibrillation and flutter in elderly. Am J Ther. 2004;11(2):95–7. https://doi.org/10.1097/00045391-200403000-00003.
19. Nair M, George LK, Koshy SK. Safety and efficacy of ibutilide in cardioversion of atrial flutter and fibrillation. J Am Board Fam Med. 2011;24(1):86–92.
20. Kahn RL, Hargett MJ, et al. Supraventricular tachyarrhythmias during total joint arthroplasty. Incidence and risk. Clin Orthop Relat Res. 1993;(296):265–9.
21. Serrano CM, Hernandez-Madrid A. Atrial fibrillation. Is it an epidemic? Rev Esp Cardiol. 2009;62(1):10–4.

Experience with MACE

6

Eric E. Harrison

Abstract

With the advent of new screening techniques and visualization platforms such as CCTA, MRI, and live video radiography, we are able to demonstrate the potential for prediction of major adverse cardiac events that has plagued our patients who have undergone major invasive joint replacement surgery. Certainly, the ability to capture bone powder during a live feed gave us the hint as to one reason how this could lead to deposition of hydroxyapatite with fibrin attachment at both ends. We have determined that this is not only a common but also a source of severe embolic events in a greater than 50% of patients. Multi-modality analysis technology with current state-of-the-art Artificial Intelligence software has tremendously helped to enhance patient care and improve patient outcomes.

Keywords

Major adverse cardiac events (MACE) · Multi-modality · Hydroxyapatite · Total hip arthroplasty (THA) · Total knee arthroplasty (TKA) · Atrial fibrillation (AF) · Paroxysmal atrial fibrillation (PAF) · Continuous Heart Rhythm Monitoring (>24 hrs) · Orthopaedic Surgery Cardiovascular Assessment Risk Score (OSCARS) · Chronic atrial fibrillation (CAF) · Left Ventricular Hypertrophy (LVH) · Pre-ventricular contractions (PVC) · Deep venous thrombosis (DVT)

E. E. Harrison (✉)
Board Chair International Cardio-Oncology Society, ICOS CEO PrivaCors Inc. Cardio-Orthopaedics®, Tampa, FL, USA

Morsani College of Medicine, University of South Florida, Tampa, FL, USA

Joint Special Operations University, Tampa, FL, USA

E. E. Harrison, N. H. Ho (eds.), *Managing Cardiovascular Risk In Elective Total Joint Arthroplasty*, https://doi.org/10.1007/978-3-031-26415-3_6

6.1 Myocardial Adverse Cardiac Events in Cardio-Orthopedics

Case Presentation: A 68-year-old Caucasian male was referred to me to assess his cardiovascular risk of total hip replacement. Twelve years ago, he presented with pericardial effusion of unknown origin treated medically and surgically with a pericardiac window. Patient had a complication of paroxysmal atrial fibrillation at that time.

In September 2017, he had a preoperative evaluation for endoscopy and recent recurrence of PAF and was referred to cardiology for preoperative evaluation for THA.

Patient was asymptomatic cardiac-wise with symptomatic hip dysfunction. There was no known history of coronary artery disease. ECG and echo were normal. He was considered low risk for TJA by several standard risk evaluations. Because of PAF, patient was started on apixaban 150 mg bid. The drug would be held 48 h before surgery. He was also started on dronedarone 400 mg bid plus ranolazine 500 mg bid. Both drugs would be given with sips of water before and after surgery to prevent PAF. The HARMONY Trial Combined Ranolazine and Dronedarone [1].

Patient had routine CCTA for evaluation of occult CAD as per our protocol. He was found to have a complex LAD plaque with a 75% obstruction. Analysis with Sherlock technology revealed a very complex lesion with a large plaque ulcer seen on 2D and 3D views (see Fig. 6.1).

Our multi-modality Sherlock Analysis from our core laboratory (Fig. 6.1) shows, by clockwise reading, the large lipid notch in the LAD with the large area of myocardium seen in blue which represents a 38% LV myocardium at risk. HeartFlow also shows vessel decreased flow seen in red. Coronary artery CT-P (CT-perfusions defects) in orange with a blue background on a polar map. Defects are seen in apical anterior and inferior basilar lateral images representing the LAD and the posterior descending arteries, with the images having a sensitivity of 85 with diffuse coronary vasodilatation caused by the contrast and adenoscan. The large well-defined plaque ulcer is seen in green in the next polar map followed by a picture of the PDA artery stenosis.

The posterior descending artery also had a 75% stenosis with a CTP (CT perfusion) defect in the inferior lateral wall.

Figure 6.2 with a manual superimposition of the myocardial CT-MPI with the echo speckle tracking strain echo with some rotation to align the images and clearly shows the same thing defects in the perfusion of the anterior wall and the inferior wall.

This patient was very similar to a patient I had 27 years prior: an elderly lady was having THA and had had a cardiac catheterization that showed a severe proximal LAD lesion with normal LV function, ECG, and echocardiogram. I was concerned about her risk of an anterior wall MI at the time of surgery and planned a TEE during THA for monitoring the wall motion of the anterior wall and the LV septum which were supplied by the diseased LAD. If during the monitoring the patient had ischemia of the anterior wall or septum, I would respond by starting IV NTG drip.

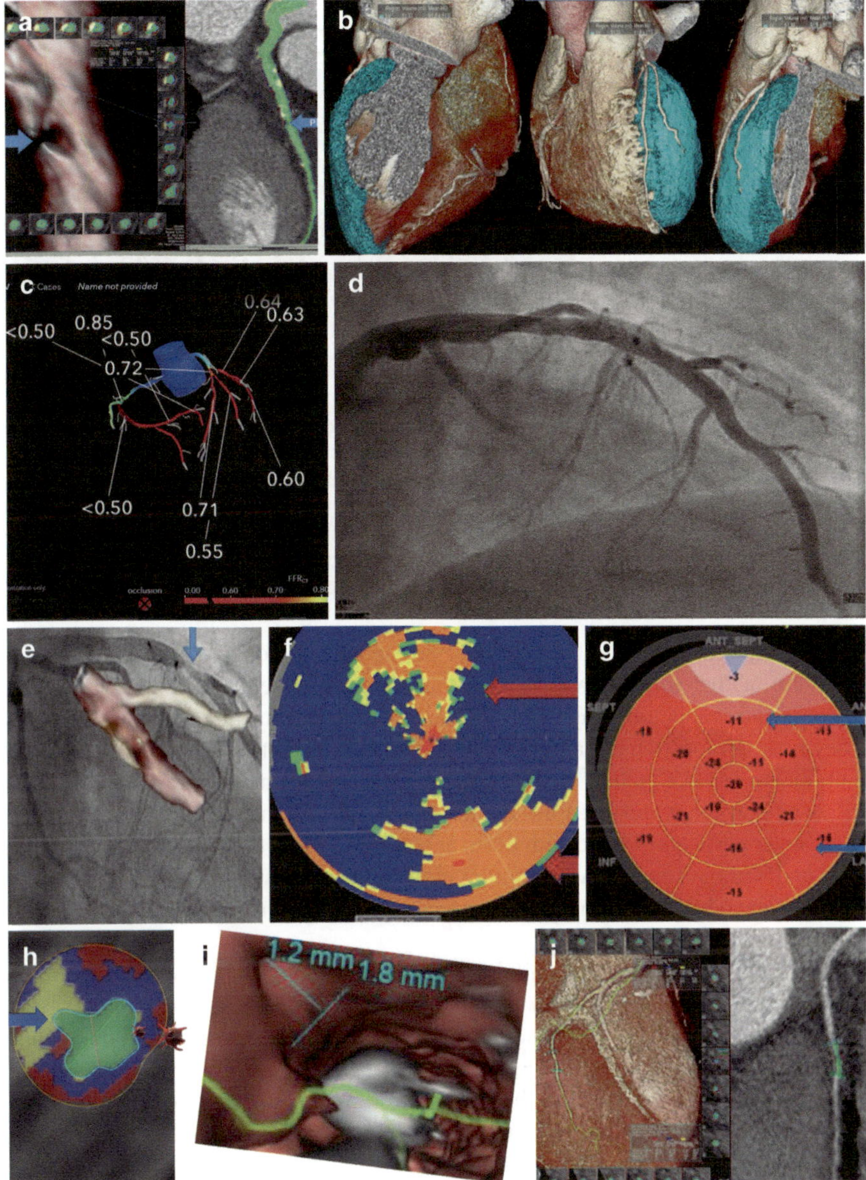

Fig. 6.1 Composite multi-modality Sherlock analysis (**a**–**j**) (not reproduced)

Surprisingly to me because of a lack of orthopedic experience, there was the sudden appearance of contrast (bone powder) in the IVC, RA, and RV while the orthopedist was hammering during hip preparation for insertion of a prothesis. The bone powder swirled about and resembled an intravenous contrast injection with dense total chamber opacification. Some people called these "snow flurries".

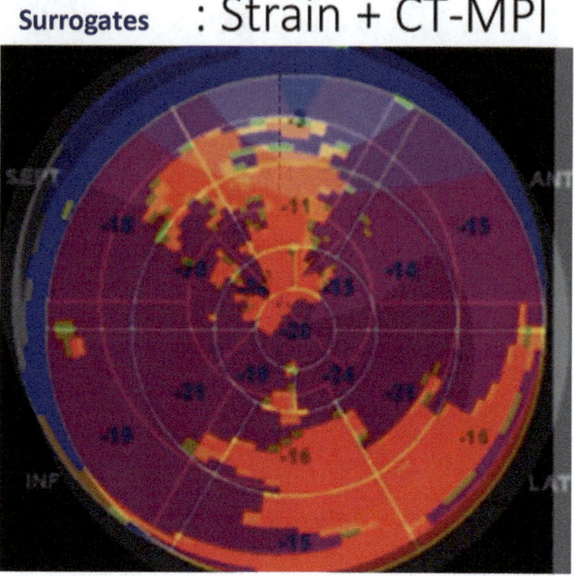

Fig. 6.2 Blood flow surrogates—strain echo overlapping with CT-MPI (not reproduced)

This appearance of the bone powder prompted a thorough investigation of the literature at that time. It was demonstrated quite frequently and was shown by microscopic evaluation to by hydroxyapatite with fibrin attachment at both ends [2]. They have demonstrated that this is not only a common but also a source of severe embolic events in a greater than 50% of patients at that time. It has been noted that the bone powder or dust was not related to cement use, marrow, fat, and consisted of granular particles of bone with fibrin at both ends. No difference between fixation with and without cement. Activation of clotting cascades was seen [3–9].

The bone powder intracardiac appearance is both seen in hip replacement as well as knee replacement.

I was able to deduce the parallels and expectations arrived at by displaying two cases with a 27-year gap and how we arrived at the prediction of a heart attack in the second patient based on the embolic risk activated by bone powder and the plaque ulcer with stenosis as a potential platelet aggregate target. Other risk factors for activating platelets in case 2 on the right picture were history of recent atrial fibrillation and the cessation of the apixaban anticoagulant for 48 h before THR, both cause more frequent thrombus generation.

Thus, we evaluated this patient further. We constructed a hypothesis based on what we found about the patient's plaques and the risk of activating platelets with bone powder release and his atrial fibrillation/cessation of anticoagulation risk of having intrinsic causes of activated platelets.

Our patient's 2D and 3D CT imaging of the LAD plaque ulcer demonstrated a 75% diameter stenosis which contains the ulcer with a convergent divergent double cone as part of the geometry of the plaque by our "Sherlock" analysis. The "bone powder" that was released from the TJA would later lead to deposition of platelets in the ulcer and result in an AWMI.

Because we demonstrated the possibility of this hypothesis, we decided to calculate the random prediction of an MI at a specific time and date. This random event occurring within 24 h after surgery in an asymptomatic patient without knowledge of his coronary anatomy was calculated as 1/150,000,000. Since we had strong anatomical factual data, we concluded he was going to have an AWMI within 24 h of his THA and would address his case accordingly. We notified his surgeon that we were going to cancel his case in the large tertiary hospital where he would be lumped with a group of 15 cases of the day. It was felt that it would be better to do his case at a small community hospital as the only case of the day by a member of the same group and where we could assign a nurse navigator to discuss the risk, follow him in the hospital closely and give him her business card cell number for contact after discharge.

The risk was explained to him in detail and that he could be followed and if the event occurred, rescued with a catheterization and stenting. He became comfortable with this proposition. He did have successful surgery as scheduled, remained on his anti-arrhythmic medications with sips of water both preoperatively and postoperatively and had an uncomplicated course and was discharged by the nurse navigator the next day at 12 noon. His daughter drove him home, settled him in, and left. He made a cup of coffee and then started having chest pain. He said he was having a heart attack as predicted and called his daughter back and called the nurse navigator who instructed him to return to the hospital ER. He had some ECG changes and slightly positive troponin. hs-Troponin-T Gen 5 Stat by Roche was already acquired and programmed by our team but every time we would order it, the insurer would deny its use even though it was less than $5.00, but they would ok the CCTA for $199. Despite the patient explaining I had predicted his heart attack, the ER doctor used the standard procedure which was to get a CT of the chest which to ruled out a PE. His CP worsened with the CT scan, the PE was ruled out, a NSTEMI was diagnosed, and he had a cardiac catheterization which revealed the LAD lesion with an area that demonstrated to have a fuzzy appearance of a clot. The area was stented with good results (Figs. 6.3 and 6.4).

The patient did not complete his infarction, had no more chest pain, his ECG returned to normal, and he was discharged home early resulting in $20,000 financial savings. Six weeks later, his cardiac MRI with gadolinium showed no heart damage (Figs. 6.5 and 6.6).

This is the first case to my knowledge of the prediction of a heart attack in an asymptomatic patient for TJA based on his CTA anatomy with a stenosis and ulcerated plaque and his potential exposure to bone powder during his TJA. He could not have preoperative stenting because he was asymptomatic and Medicare would not pay for it. Thus, we followed him with a nurse navigator and took action after THA when he became symptomatic from myocardial ischemia and elevated his troponin.

This is a good time to review the other cases that we encountered in our CCTAs in our TJA acquired data base involving the majority of the TJA patients. Those TJA patients who did not have CCTA were those allergic to contrast, those with significant chronic kidney disease (they got a calcium score), those who had chronic atrial fibrillation, flutter, or tachyarrhythmia, patients with prior recent cardiac

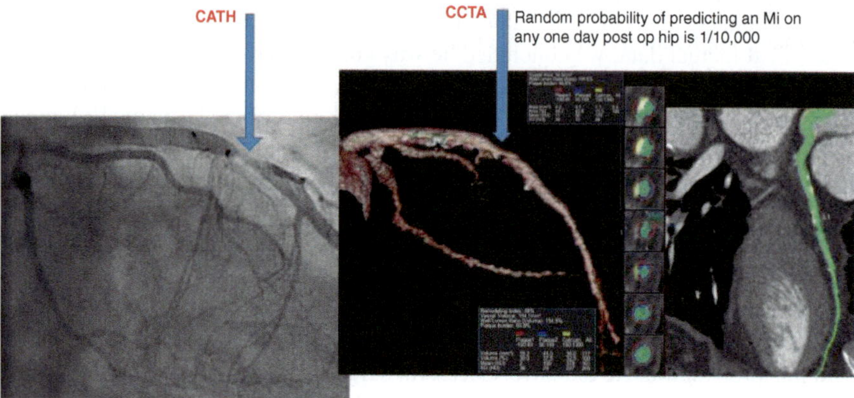

Fig. 6.3 This slide shows the cardiac catheterization anatomical imaging with a fuzzy area at the LAD convergent divergent double cone stenotic plaque site. The other two images are the earlier diagnostic CT showing the complex LAD stenosis, plaque, and ulcer

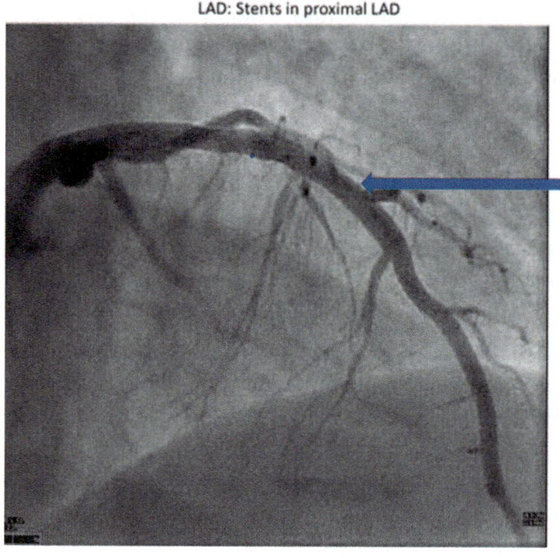

Fig. 6.4 The arrow is pointing to a normal appearing LAD after stenting (not reproduced)

catheterization, and patients who simply declined. Those who did have the procedure have been scored by a CCTA score developed by the SCCT and is an open source. CT Coronary Angiography: "CAD-RADSTM Coronary Artery Disease e Reporting and Data System" posted on November 26, 2017 by admin. **The CAD-RADS scoring system** is a reporting system for rating the extent of coronary artery disease and is used internationally by advanced imaging physicians to standardize the classification of the coronary atherosclerotic disease so that all are expressing

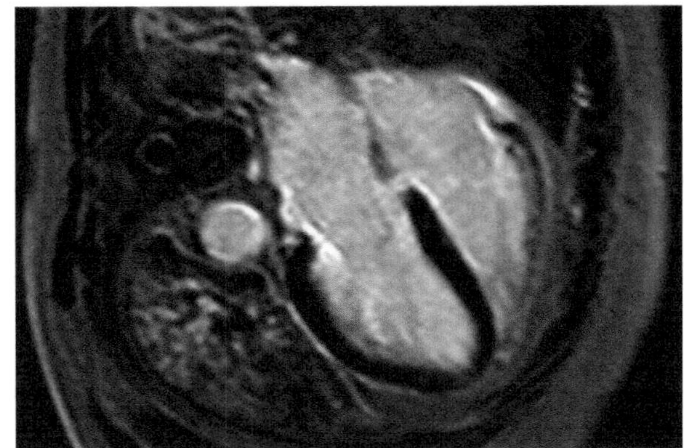

Fig. 6.5 Normal late gadolinium cardiac MRI showing no scar (not reproduced)

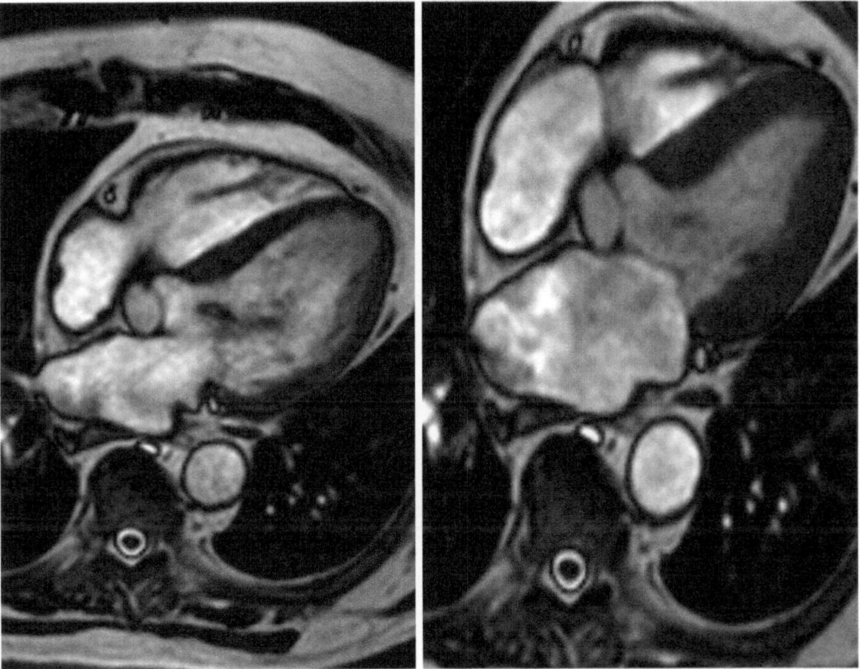

Fig. 6.6 Normal LV contractility on cardiac MRI (not reproduced)

the same data to one another [10]. Please refer to this chart as you read out interpretations. We also use our own data that we have accumulated with our application of the app Sherlock developed at the time of association with IBM Watson (Table 6.1).

With these factors in mind, I will show you the data we generated on our first group of 87 TJA patients. Eighty seven patients having their CCTA and the arteries classified according to our CCTA data system and our Sherlock application showed up with this picture (Fig. 6.7). As with OSCARS, we have a reducible risk score for coronary arteries that begins with high risk and is modified by our planned protocol

Table 6.1 Our Sherlock application developed as we gained years of experience starting in 2004 on 16 slice imaging and continuing uninterrupted for 17 years as Vital Images and now Canon licensed investigators who have trained many cardiac fellows in this program

Plaque anatomy characteristics on CCTA	
(1) Percent diameter stenosis	**accurate patient-specific geometric models**
(2) Percent necrotic core <50 Hu	**and physiological boundary conditions**
(3) Distance & pointing of necrotic core to closest lumen	
(4) LV thickness/mass	
(5) Diastolic blood pressure	
(6) Traditional spotty calcification, napkin ring	
(7) Convergent/Divergent double cone	
(8) Angle and length of convergent Axial Plaque Strain (APS) WSS is Minimal	**:18% angle greatest thrust**
(9) Angle and length of divergence	
(10) Heart flow parameters ΔP	
(11) Peak velocity	
(12) Solubility of CO_2 at various temperature, vapor pressure > wall pressure	
(13) Length of narrowest point	
(14) Density ratio of narrowest contrast, least dense/max dense point distally?	
(15) Elasticity of the artery	
(16) Distal coronary calcified plaque	**Reflective wave?**
(17) Proximity to origin	
(18) Radius gradient (radius change over length)	
(19) Plaque internal surface area	
(20) Plaque area of greatest stenosis	
(21) Retrograde vs. antegrade flow	

100s of plaque characteristics can be analyzed for correlation by Al and validation by application to a different data set

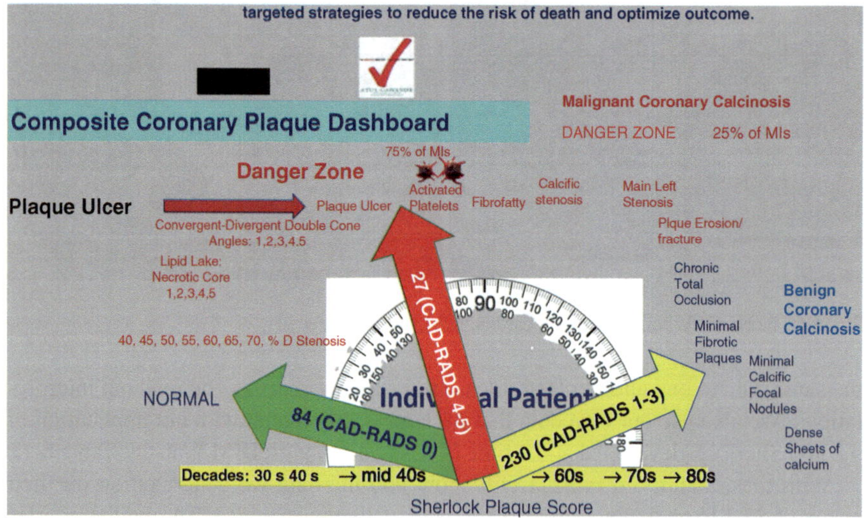

Fig. 6.7 This slide shows the unadjusted findings in our group of TJA patients who had 314 CCTAs. Green: no CAD 84, Yellow: CAD-RADs 1-3 low risk too, and Red: High risk of 27 which need to be adjudicated with the Sherlock application by intuitive cardiologists

which considered plaques only risky with an ulcerated plaque! We initially classified the patients according to the risk that they showed from the data system and Sherlock together. Twenty four patients had no risk of atherosclerotic coronary artery disease in that there was zero calcium score and no observable coronary plaque on the Canon workstation and by the use of our Sherlock application. These patients were classified immediately as green. CAR-RADS 1–3 was classified as intermediate risk (yellow) were reclassified for TJA as low risk (green) and joined the green group bringing it up to 24 + 50 = 74. Those who clearly had CAD with stents or CABGs were reclassified if they had patent stents or patent grafts that establish rerouting of blood supply in those with stenosis or occlusive disease. These were 9 which gave us now a total of 24 + 50 + 9 = 83.Those four who were classified as high risk (red) were examined in detail and three were reclassified as low risk (green) for TJA which is considered an intermediate risk procedure by the AHA/ACC guidelines. This brought the low-risk total to 83. Of these three patients over 65 years old, one of these patients had moderate in several vessels which were stented and had a CTO of the OM1 with ischemia which was not stented. Stenting 60% lesions and not stenting the 100% DM CTO which showed ischemia was a useless exercise that delayed his TJA. His surgery was delayed 6 months until he could be taken off of dual antiplatelet therapy which was a problem he had to tolerate by using a walker and enduring considerable pain. Another had a LAD 76% stenosis without symptoms but was inactive because of her knee pain which limited her tolerance to exercise. The third patient had a chemical stress test that was positive in the wrong distribution and had an RCA that had an ectopic high takeoff origin and although the interventional cardiologists showed a great deal of effort for hours several times, they were unable to engage the orifice of the vessel with the convention catheters they used so they canceled the patient for TKA because of their binary decision to delay surgery because they couldn't get to the area to stent. I felt she would not have symptoms from a 50–70% RCA lesion with HeartFlow reduction of flow that was only intermediate (74%). That became true until after she had TKA and started developing dyspnea on exertion during physical therapy and was sent to Dr. Paolo Angelini in Houston for use of the Angelini catheter which immediately engaged the high RCA and she was stented in 5 min. Thus, the patient did not need the pre-TJA stent to have her surgery. So much for binary decision-making as being a reason to delay TJA.

That last red high risk patient who is the case we presented above and he remained high risk with a nurse navigator assigned to follow him throughout the perioperative period because of his risk of an MI and he did have a postoperative NSTEMI within 24 h of his surgery which was forecast by our Sherlock risk factors of decreased perfusion of the myocardial CT, and the presence of a plaque ulcer and a stenotic LAD with convergent divergent double cones, and the theoretical exposure to bone powder.

Our teams initially classified risk by the plaque system combined with our Sherlock application, which contributed to the reducible risk of our 86 cases; only one remained in the red as high risk.

Our TJA patients that had CCTA: 341 total with 84 being no risk because of no calcium in the coronaries and no plaque. 230 were our initially intermediate risk because of CAD-RADs 1–3 and 27 CAD-RADs 4-5 which were colored red. All of the yellow were reclassified as low risk green:84 + 230 = 314. These that are depicted red have not been reclassified according to our system and our Sherlock application and were carefully adjudicated on a case-by-case basis. Some have been turned down for elective surgery; one patient with two occluded grafts was turned down for THA by three cardiologists. The patient had become wheelchair bound and was desperate for the surgery. Upon review, the occluded grafts had become occluded because they went to patent vessels with minimal CAD! Just drilling deep gave me the information to authorize THA and free him from a wheelchair life. Unfortunately, cardiologists don't have the leisure time to drill deep because they are so besieged by administrators to deliver more billable RVUs for them. The high risk patients were reclassified with one patient continued as red because of a plaque with an ulcer but no significant obstruction. This patient was navigated and did well. Sherlock tells me to ignore the plaques unless there is significant coronary obstructive plaque. Both have to be present (Fig. 6.7).

The high risk patients who are reclassified are followed after surgery for any event that they develop in 90 days if bundled. Their primary doctor is also alerted. If they have an interventional cardiologist, it seems that he is on alert for making binary stent decisions and seems to not get involved with cases that are complex cardiovascular cases that involve hypertension, LVH, PAF, TIAs, or other medical problems that are very important in this patient group. Non-interventionalist cardiologists go on the defensive when discussing the OSCARs to rely on the anatomy when making decisions and to err on the conservative side when deciding how to treat and whether medical or interventional. The only interventional case we had was the lady with the abdominal aortic aneurysm whom we had acquire an endovascular stent but TJA surgery did proceed according to when it was scheduled.

One result was of interest that 25 patients were readmitted to the service within 90 days with 22 having only preoperative ECGs and three having an EKG and echo. During this period of bundling, our group had three admissions: The NSTEMI (we predicted whom we saved $20,000 on), a patient in chronic AF (who received more calcium channel blocked by her primary care doctor and was admitted for AF bradycardia), and a gentleman that was outside of the 90 day period who was readmitted with a SVT.

Our patient had had delayed surgery because of stenting the RCA (moderate stenosis) (Fig. 6.8) and second OM2 (moderate stenosis) but no stenting of the CTO ischemic OM1 (Fig. 6.9) came to the ER with back pain, a positive troponin was discovered, and he had a catheterization which mistakenly identified a stenotic vessel in the LAD which the operator thought had been stented (contrary to the EMR and data) and sent him to surgery for CABG by mistake. This resulted in a prolonged recovery in the rehabilitation center adjacent to the hospital.

Patients in this group sometimes were bundled with cohorts under the CMS national bundling program which ran a limiting time span (ending it, ending the bundling cohort and comparison) that could be compared to them because of a

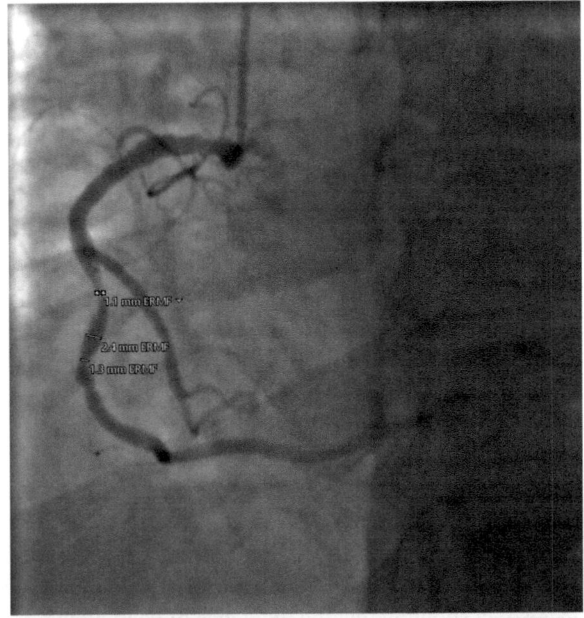

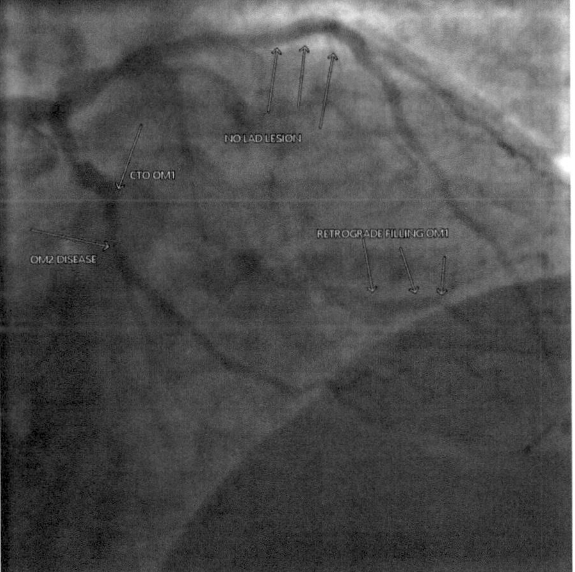

Figs. 6.8 and 6.9 These slides show the patient lesions as moderate in both the RCA which became stented later on this cine and the OM2 which also was stented on this cine but no stenting of the ischemic muscle of CTO OM1 or LAD stenting which was thought to have been stented by the interventionist who did the last catheterization

match of complexity and a lack of these tests by other cardiologists in the group. To further define this, we are choosing a large cohort with equal identity but different orthopedists in the group and will publish this data after it is assembled.

We also scored the carotids ultrasound for obstruction or plaque and found none in our large group of patients. I initially thought carotid disease would be the cause of CVAs/TIAs but was very surprised that the cause was PAF in our group of patients. We also searched for internal carotid plaque ulcers but did not find any in this patient group. They are best searched for with CT of the carotids with application of Vital Images SurePlaque (Fig. 6.10).

Now is a good time to review that current medical literature to see how this has progressed in cardio-orthopedics. In 1983, as an invasive cardiologist, I wrote a chapter in "Noncardiac Surgery in the Cardiac Patient" Stephen P. Glasser MD, Futura Publishing Company, Mount Kisco, New York. At that time, there were no prospective angiographic studies of patients in anticipation of noncardiac surgery and I could only find one retrospective report.

Since then, there has been some review of the finding of cardiac catheterization prior to noncardiac surgery in the National Cardiovascular Data Registry (NCDR) CathPCI Registry. This was a very large group of 194,444 patients. Those found with obstructive disease were treated by intervention or medical therapy about equally even though this does not follow guidelines [11].

However, I cannot find a group of patients having a cardiac catheterization at a single institution prior to TJA nor can I find a group having CCTA prior to TJA.

We can find observations concluded after TJA which may be an opportunity to reflect. However, post hoc ergo propter hoc isn't always valid. Dr. Leonard S. Sommer (1924–2020) of the University of Miami School of Medicine published an abstract showing that the incidence of heart attack 24 h after catheterization is the same as the incidence preoperatively 24 h before the cath. That is because many patients are getting cardiac cath because of unstable angina. This was before the PTCA/Stents. Only those with ostial main left disease might have obstruction by the catheter during the procedure which would accelerate their ischemia resulting in demise 30 min later. All the others were fairly unchanged. We'll have to keep this in mind when reviewing the postoperative TJA literature.

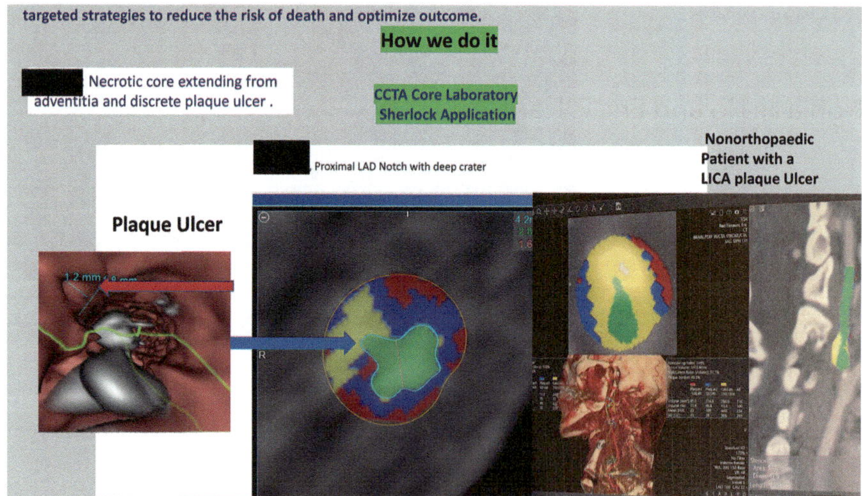

Fig. 6.10 Shows the coronary plaque ulcer presented in our case report in this chapter and contrasted to it is an internal carotid ulcer shown on the right with application of SUREPLAQUE

Thus, a retrospective study was constructed to review 4,323,045 patients who had surgery in the hospital from 2008–2012 with identification of preoperative comorbidities and correlating them to congestive heart failure, valvular heart disease, and COPD in declining rate of morbidity [12].

You might ask what was the rate of morbidity and mortality preoperatively? In the study of one prospective controlled group and the rest retrospective [13], there were no myocardial infarction or specific arrhythmias specially assessed!

JA Singh and his group studied "Cardiac and thromboembolic complications and mortality in patients undergoing total hip and total knee arthroplasty." From 1994 to 2008 at Mayo Clinic in Rochester, NY, showed post-operative cardiovascular complications with morbidity and mortality of 13.8% and 13.4% of those over 65 years old with assessment of 90 occurrence and predictors of cardiac complications all based on history and retrospective data but without anatomical information and no comparison of a similar groups risk 90 days before surgery or a group without surgery and their complications over 90 days (Table 6.2), with the finding of 90-day cardiac events in THA and TKA of 6.8%, an example that some people in this age group have with mixed results of CHF, MI, or arrhythmias which is a mixed bag of different anatomical origin which was not clear. Anatomically, we could separate out those with PAF, CHF from LVH and HTN, the possibility of MINS elevation of postop cardiac markers but all predictive anatomically preoperatively all predicated on our OSCAR score of being lower with treatment for 30 days reducing the risk! Consequently, our 90 complication rate was our index patient with a predicted MI in 24 h and the patient with chronic atrial fibrillation that developed a bradycardia due to her primary care doctor upwardly adjusting her rate control medications was 2/430 = 0.46% compared to those numbers acquired in Olmstead County. Arrhythmias were the largest number of complications of the three possible cardiac complications of myocardial infarction, arrhythmias, and congestive heart failure.

Table 6.2 All cardiac risk was low for first 30 days but grew higher at 90 days and was based on history rather than anatomy (OSCARs) and the Charlson Score designed for epidemiology was used for retroactive risk score assessment

Singh, JA et al. Mayo 2011						
7-Day		30-Day		90-Day		
THA (*n* = 1195) *n* (%)	TKA (*n* = 1604) *n* (%)	THA (*n* = 1195) *n* (%)	TKA (*n* = 1604) *n* (%)	THA (*n* = 1195) *n* (%)	TKA (*n* = 1604) *n* (%)	
All cardiac events	29 (2.4%)	33 (2.1%)	61 (5.1%)	85 (5.3%)	14.8% >65	108 (6.7%)
Myocardial infarction	3 (0.3%)	2 (0.1%)	11 (0.9%)	14 (0.9%)	14 (1.2%)	22 (2.8% >65)
Arrhythmia	28 (2.3%)	26 (1.6%)	41 (3.4%)	65 (4.0%)	57 (4.8%)	83 (10.4% >65)
Congestive heart failure	8 (0.7%)	7 (0.4%)	23 (1.9%)	24 (1.5%)	32 (2.7%)	32 (4% >65)
Olmsted county residents mean ± SD or *n* (%)						
		THA (*n* = 1195 patients)			TKA (*n* = 1608 patients)	
Age		66.6 ± 13.1			68.1 ± 10.6	

If we look at that arrhythmias group alone, we find a 90-day rate of 4.8% for elective THA and a 90-day rate for elective TKA of 5.2%. I suspect this means new onset arrhythmia. We had no patients with new onset arrhythmias which gives us a 0.0%. As you know, all patients at 30 days prior to surgery with a preoperative history of palpitations, HTN, finding of HTN, finding of LVH of 13 or greater, evidence of a large LA, ECG evidence of AF, significant MR, were monitor by a Continuous Heart Rhythm recorder for variable lengths of time for PAF or Flutter and any other arrhythmias and those with PAF or Flutter were started on a DOAC and also if not on an anti-arrhythmias ranolazine 500 mg bid and dronedarone 400 mg bid which were maintained with sips of water on their operative day with a 48 h hold on the DOAC.

The next most common cardiac was CHF with 2.7% for THA and 2.0 for TKA. We had one patient who came out of the ER with uncontrolled HTN and CHF which had been missed on our check list from our echo group of LVH (13 mm) patients who would have been monitored for therapeutic BP control and if not under control, an additional drug would have been added. No other patients had CHF in 90 days.

The third and least complication was myocardial infarction which were 1.2% for THA and 1.4% for TKA. Our only case of myocardial infarction was the NSTEMI that we predicted was going to have a cardiac event because of his LAD anatomy which consisted of a 75% lesion with a plaque ulcer with a convert-divergent double cone. The myocardial infarction rate was then 1/430 = 0.23%, lower than the experience in in Olmstead years ago.

I'm not sure what this means but could have quite a few possibilities but the fact that it closed out over 13 years ago means it is less meaningful because so much has changed in cardiology; Knee and Hip Replacements Linked to Heart Attacks, Older Age, Recent Heart Attacks Increased the Risks Associated With Joint Replacement Surgeries. They said that heart attacks were 25 times and 30 times more common in patients having hip or knee surgery, respectively. So much has changed from statin therapy for elevated cholesterol to the administration of aspirin in postoperative TJA. Patients now have one-third of the cardiac events that they used to have in all study groups [14].

Another study showed a perioperative patient support system was unable to mitigate the risk of hospital readmission for total hip arthroplasty patients with High American Society of Anesthesiologists Grades. This program with an RN engaged Navigator did not lower the risk of readmission raises issues of the diagnosis and treatment of this complicated group of patients specifically to control of blood pressure/HTN/LVH/CHF, prevention of PAF and TIA/CVA, lowering cholesterol to mitigate CAD, preventing DVT/PE, and watching for aortic dilatation [10, 15].

Certainly, the separation of medical silos prevents the integration of these complex medical fields in solving interrelated problems that coexist and prevent obvious solutions advanced in our careful observation of this group of patients that I had cared for myself and failed to address their obvious problems. It is hoped that the anatomical identification preoperatively with OSCARs will give us the option of treating this group for 30 days before surgery to prevent these comorbidity complications but any other complications that could occur in 90 days and then thereafter as we did with the people with HTN/LVH/CHF, PAF/TIAs/CVAs, CAD/STEMI/NSTEMI, DVT/PE, dilated aorta, and moderate to severe aortic stenosis. It seems that we have solved these problems by bridging silos whether its cardio-oncology, cardio-neurology, cardio-diabetes, and now cardio-orthopedics and assigning the referred more complicated and older patients to a cardio-orthopedist who is committed to a very careful evaluation 30 days before surgery by applying the OSCARs by echocardiogram, carotid and aortic U/S and CCTA and using the score for decided further testing and treatment which can reduce the score before surgery. Those with significant CAD by CAD-RADs and SHERLOCK analysis are carefully evaluated and not stented since they are asymptomatic. They are also followed after surgery. These did not have any complications during the 90 days except the one with the lesion in the RCA with a high take who had DOE during PT as expected and was sent to Dr. Angelini for Angelini catheter stenting of the RAC.

As far as thromboembolism goes, all of these were detected by the CCTAs, TJA was cancelled and patients were treated medically and later sent to surgery without subsequent problems. Patients who had a history of DVT or PE in the past but had no emboli on CCTA, received enoxaparin postoperatively by guidelines and had no complications.

References

1. Reiffel JA, Camm AJ, Belardinelli L, et al. The HARMONY trial: combined ranolazine and dronedarone in the management of paroxysmal atrial fibrillation: mechanistic and therapeutic synergism. Circ Arrhythm Electrophysiol. 2015;8(5):1048–56.
2. Hagio K, Sugano N, Takashina M, et al. Embolic events during total hip arthroplasty: an echocardiographic study. J Arthroplast. 2003;18:186–92.
3. Hayakawa M, Fujioka Y, Morimoto Y, et al. Pathological evaluation of venous emboli during total hip arthroplasty. Anaesthesia. 2001;56(6):571–5.
4. Christie J, Burnett R, Potts HR, Pell AC. Echocardiography of transatrial embolism during cemented and uncemented hemiarthroplasty of the hip. J Bone Joint Surg Br. 1994;76(3):409–12.
5. Lafont ND, Kostucki WM, Marchand PH, Michaux MN, Boogaerts JG. Embolism detected by transoesophageal echocardiography during hip arthroplasty. Can J Anaesth. 1994;41(9):850–3.
6. Bisignani G, Bisignani M, Pasquale GS, Greco F. Intraoperative embolism and hip arthroplasty: intraoperative transesophageal echocardiographic study. J Cardiovasc Med (Hagerstown). 2008;9(3):277–81.
7. Koessler MJ, Pitto RP. Fat and bone marrow embolism in total hip arthroplasty. Acta Orthop Belg. 2001;67(2):97–109.
8. Dambrosio M, Tullo L, Moretti B, et al. Hemodynamic and respiratory changes during hip and knee arthroplasty. An echocardiographic study. Anestesiol. 2002;68(6):537–47.
9. Christie J, Robinson CM, Pell AC, McBirnie J, Burnett R. Transcardiac echocardiography during invasive intramedullary procedures. Bone Joint Surg Br. 1995;77(3):450–5.
10. Foldyna B, Szilveszter B, Scholtz JE, et al. CAD-RADS—a new clinical decision support tool for coronary computed tomography angiography. Eur Radiol. 2018;28(4):1365–72.
11. Schulman-Marcus J, Feldman DN, Rao SV, et al. Characteristics of patients undergoing cardiac catheterization before noncardiac surgery: a report from the National Cardiovascular Data Registry CathPCI registry. JAMA Intern Med. 2016;176(5):611–8.

12. Hustedt JW, Goltzer O, Bohl DD, et al. Calculating the cost and risk of comorbidities in Total joint arthroplasty in the United States. J Arthroplast. 2017;32(2):355–361.e1.
13. Xu J, Cao JY, Chaggar GS, Negus JJ. Comparison of outpatient versus inpatient total hip and knee arthroplasty: a systematic review and meta-analysis of complications. J Orthop. 2019;17:38–43.
14. Lalmohamed A, Vestergaard P, Klop C, et al. Timing of acute myocardial infarction in patients undergoing Total hip or knee replacement—a Nationwide cohort study. Arch Intern Med. 2012;172(16):1229–35.
15. Woittiez KJ, Noble JL. Respiratory failure after Total hip replacement. J Intensive & Crit Care. 2016;2(4):43–5.

Risk Evaluation

7

Eric E. Harrison

Abstract

This chapter introduces by way of case review, anecdotal evidence and evidence-based experience, the need for closer cooperation between orthopedics and cardiology, particularly in relation to total joint arthroplasty (TJA). The use of computerized axial tomography scans (CT scans) is recommended as a preoperative diagnostic tool along with echocardiography. The rationale for the use of noninvasive cardiac imaging is explained, and the necessity for a comprehensive workup vis-a-vis cardio-orthopedics is justified by our observational comparison readmission rate before and after the institution of cardiac imaging prior to surgery.

Keywords

Cardio-orthopedics · Total joint arthroplasty (TJA) · Preoperative evaluation · Cardiac risk of TJA · Perioperative risk assessment

There is a growing need for hip and knee replacement surgery as the aging population grows and as sophisticated treatment with TJA develops into the ability to maintain patient functional capacity in modern mature advanced developed world countries. This is accelerated by many people becoming overweight as they age. Estimations of projected volume are increasing dramatically as the population of aging individuals grows in our society.

E. E. Harrison (✉)
Board Chair International Cardio-Oncology Society, ICOS CEO PrivaCors Inc. Cardio-Orthopaedics®, Tampa, FL, USA

Morsani College of Medicine, University of South Florida, Tampa, FL, USA

Joint Special Operations University, Tampa, FL, USA

E. E. Harrison, N. H. Ho (eds.), *Managing Cardiovascular Risk In Elective Total Joint Arthroplasty*, https://doi.org/10.1007/978-3-031-26415-3_7

There are many factors involved with life style restricted by various levels of inactivity from having prolonged osteoarthritis ranging from a limp to disability with the use of a walker which may evolve over a period of years. Over this time, it is seen as developing into obesity including metabolic syndrome, visceral fat deposits, and diabetes but also the osteoarthritis developing into chronic inflammation and the use of NSAIDS: all of these factors are active in contributing to coronary artery disease, MACE, low EF → CHF, hypertension with LVH, atrial fibrillation with TIAs and CVAs, activated platelets with DVT/PE, and sleep apnea.

By 2030 more than 570,000 THA procedures will be performed annually in the USA, representing 175% increase from 2005 volume as well as more than 3.5 million Total Knee Arthroplasty (TKA) cases are estimated to be completed each year, a staggering 673% increase. This will raise Medicare's TJA spending to an estimated $50 billion annually.

Pre-surgical period is often proceeded by years of osteoarthritis, inflammation, NSAID use, sedentary life style, obesity, DM, metabolic syndrome, and visceral fat accumulation. This is known to increase in cardiovascular event risk. 0–6 months post-surgery has increased risk of activation of clotting factors, leading to greatly increased but declining risk of MI. One-year post-TJA will show increased physical activity leading to weight loss and decline in metabolic syndrome, resulting in decreased risk of cardiac event.

Obviously, these parameters of the absence of exercise, the presence of inflammation, and changes in metabolism are going to change these patients risk profiles over time, and they may acquire these additional diseases that they did not have before. If they did not have primary care doctors, the patient won't know this. If they do have primary care doctors, the doctors may not have discovered these insidious changes on a once-a-year visit or if the doctors are in the NHS, the yearly assessment visit may have been eliminated to open more slots for those with new onset symptoms rather than silent disease onset.

With this in mind, let's review the AAOS guidelines which unfortunately include only one non-orthopedic medical complication, preventing venous thromboembolic disease in patients undergoing elective TJA with 850 pages of guidelines [1]. With these guidelines and an alertness for these complications, of our 430 patients, 3 had pulmonary emboli discovered preoperatively on their routine CCTAs. There is also aggressive treatment postoperatively where we had no pulmonary emboli arise.

Now that cardiovascular disease is the primary non-orthopedic complication in elective TJA, it will be a good idea to openly list these guidelines since listing the thromboembolic disease guidelines has been so effective.

Let's see what cardiovascular guidelines have been listed for total knee or hip replacement:

- Patients were asked if they had a history of DVT, PE, MI, arrhythmia, or stroke.
- In patients with known CAD or new onset symptoms or asymptomatic over 50 years of age, a more extensive history and physical is recommended and preoperative evaluation tailored to the individual [2].

Because of these warnings on patients over 50, the multiple risk factors these patients incur during osteoarthritis, it was felt by our group that they would like the history of symptoms because of inactivity and disability from lack of ambulation. This led us to the prediction of risk from an anatomical rather than a historical review. It would be helpful to include chemical biomarkers with the anatomical ones, and despite having established the Roche V troponin T platform, we were not able to get beyond insurance denial of the chemical biomarkers but not the expensive anatomical ones.

The elevated troponin postoperatively in 13.5% of TJA patients is of great concern as what it means in terms of MINS (Myocardial Injury after Non-Cardiac Surgery). Is this from coronary artery-driven myocardial ischemia or from myocardial oxygen demand versus noncoronary nonobstructive supply which can be caused by some of the factors we found so prevalent such as rapid paroxysmal atrial fibrillation, left ventricular hypertrophy with hypertension, perhaps OSA, pulmonary emboli, and other possible embolic events.

The American Academy of Orthopaedic Surgery has put together their own guideline for TJA. These AAOS guidelines include 183 pages about PE and DVT guidelines, and two pages of guidelines for MI. The huge gap in AAOS guidelines. Elective hip and knee cardiac complication rates are high, yet, still are not addressed in AAOS guidelines. Cardiac complication rates of all ages compose of 13–20% postoperative positive troponins. One out of seven patients with a cardiac history have cardiovascular complications. Cardiovascular complications have taken the lead as thromboembolic complications are almost eliminated. Perhaps as these cardiovascular risks are so well illustrated by OSCARs, an anatomical risk score, which is well identified just as the orthopedic structure has been identified anatomically in the same way, this may easily be inserted into these guidelines. This is very useful in preventing cardiovascular complications in patients over 65 years old undergoing elective hip and knee arthroplasty.

Findings published in the Journal of Surgical Research concluded patients with a history of coronary artery disease undergoing TJA were at higher risk for adverse cardiac events. "Based on the findings of this study, it appears that there is no increased risk of in-hospital mortality and complications (except for myocardial infarction) in patients with a history of coronary artery revascularization undergoing TJA. We also found perioperative cardiac arrhythmia, particularly atrial fibrillation, to be an independent predictor of in-hospital adverse events" (Fig. 7.1) [3].

There is still concern for myocardial infarction in patients having CABG followed eventually by TJA. There was concern and cancelation of two of our study patients: one was cancelled for TJA because of two closed CABG SVGs which bypassed coronaries with only 40% lesions. We okayed the surgery which was performed without complications. The other patient had an aberrant right coronary which came off high and could not reached with two catheterizations. That patient had been screened by a pharmacological nuclear scan that showed a defect in the wrong anatomical distribution. She also was okayed for TJA and had no problems until she was in rehabilitation and developed shortness of breath during exertion.

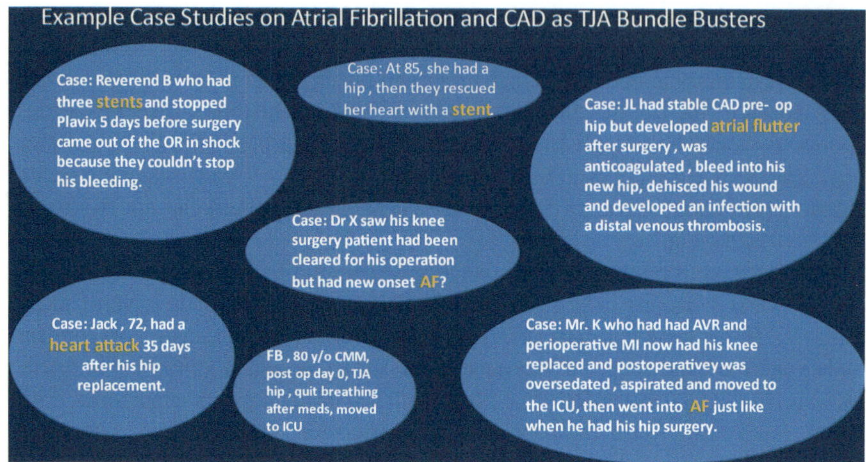

Fig. 7.1 Our curation of our data base display of the TJA prompted us to do this study (not reproduced)

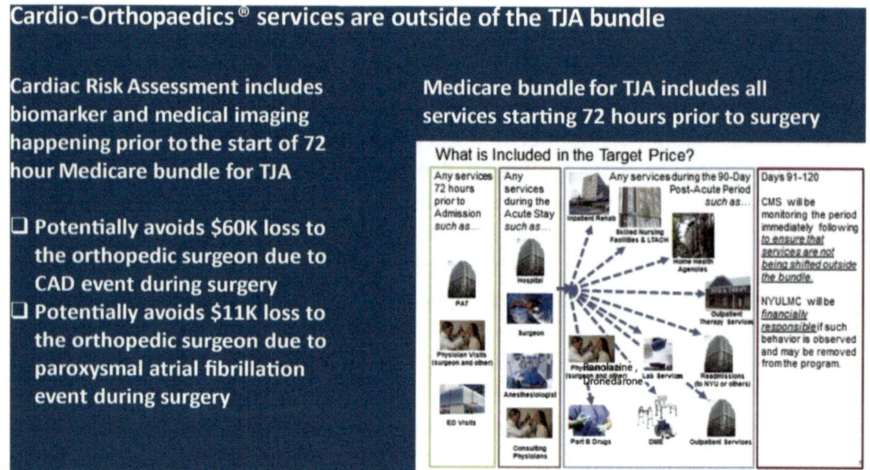

Fig. 7.2 A formulation of Cardio-Orthopedics could be considered as a Pre-bundling Actionable Pre-symptomatic advanced Cardiac Evaluation with Imaging for recognition and prevention of Major Adverse Medical Events after TJA in CJR payment models—a heuristic model (not reproduced)

She was sent to Dr. Paolo Angelini, who put a stent in the RCA using the Angelini catheter designed for that access.

Data collection registry for the TJA/CAD/AF being built by PRIVACORS and the Florida Orthopaedic Institute to advance bundle busters (Fig. 7.2). Setting guidelines to:

- Readmissions in 30, 60, 90 days
- Cost of program

- Cost reduction of bundled cases
- Risk Prediction
  - Initial risk score
  - Attenuated risk score by personal precision protocol
- Projected long-term cardiac risk reduction from imaging used in the cardio-orthopedic model
- Construct new orthopedic guidelines for CAD/PAF

With these thoughts in mind, we would like to present two representative cases the first one prior to the start of our study of the anatomy of patients for TJA and the second case after and inclusive in our study to see how they score by various risk scores used traditionally for preoperative evaluation and how they will compare to a new anatomical scoring system which can look to very specific areas that may give a better predictor of immediate postoperative cardiac complications but may also be predictive of long-term medical management and possible prolongation of life after TJA.

7.1 Case 1

JL is 77 years old who has known CAD with a totally occluded LAD and PTCA/stenting of the D1. He has an antero-apical area of endocardial calcification. There is no evidence of progressive CAD involving the LCX and the RCA. He has a history of obesity, DM, HTN and OSA. He had prior THA 8 years prior and was scheduled for LHA. Echocardiogram showed an EF of 40%. This case preceded our use of cardio-Orthopedics and was a good example of the reason to estimate his risk score anatomically.

He proceeded to THA only to have a complicated course first with atrial flutter, anticoagulation, wound bleeding with dehiscence, infection, DVT, and continued antibiotic therapy indefinitely. This case alerted our team to unexpected cardiovascular complications that might be prevented with preoperative assessment such as monitoring for PAF and looking for LAE prior to surgery in someone with a very complicated cardiac history who had arrived at a continued stable course that had potential to be upended by TJA. With early discovery of PAF and preventive preoperative treatment with dronedarone and ranolazine continuing into surgery with the medications given wit sips of water on the day of surgery this cascade of events might have been avoided. If that was not the case, and atrial flutter arose postoperatively, then rapid early COVERT cardioversion might have been the way to avoid the need for anticoagulation therapy and sequelae (See chapter on PAF recognition and prevention). The guidelines for the COVERT cardioversion experiment from Finland are inserted in the slide here below.

7.2 Before Cardio-Orthopedics

Example 1: The Case of "Jo Lar"

- 77 years old MWM with R hip replacement in 8 years ago without problems now presents for L hip replacement.
- Acute AWMI 1984 with LAD occlusion with PTCA. Recurrent event 1993 with LAD atherectomy. 1993 PTCA of D1.
- Last CCTA 2014 (no change from 2005) showed no progressive CAD, large area of AW hypokinesis with calcification of the subendocardium with EF stable at 40% with normal LA and mild MR 2/04/14. Hx of Bilateral LE lymphedema, saphenous vein ablation L in past. C/O DOE, Hx of HTN, DM, OSA.
- Cardiology "stable and low risk?"
- Surgery: L hip replaced
- Post-op atrial flutter → Hep Anticoagulation 9 days post-op wound bleeding and dehiscence, readmission, I & D surgery with multiple antibiotic Rx for infection.
- DVT L lower extremity with Rx coumadin.
- Coumadin to be continued × 6 months and doxycycline indefinitely. Rehab delayed. Total Cost: $ 39,934.83 ($21,000 over).
- Cardiologist thinking at the time: "Treat the heart, don't worry about the hip."

The study from Finland encourages the cardioversion to proceed before 12 h elapses to prevent pulmonary emboli which can develop after 12 h. This made timing of utmost importance. Our group prefers cardioversion with CORVERT versus electrical cardioversion to avoid the patient immediate post shock sudden muscle contraction with vigorous motion which may dislodge the recently implanted hip or knee prothesis:

- Researchers from Finland studied 2481 patients who underwent 5116 successful cardioversions from 2003 to 2010. These patients had AF of less than 48 h and were not on anticoagulation. The research team then retrospectively reviewed their medical records looking for post-cardioversion thromboembolic events. To determine the importance of timing of cardioversion from the onset of symptoms, the researchers compared three groups of patients: those cardioverted within 12 h of onset ($n = 2440$), between 12 and 24 h ($n = 1840$), and between 24 and 48 h ($n = 836$).
- They reported 38 thromboembolic events in 38 patients (0.7% overall incidence), with eight events (0.3%) in the <12-h group (was this really 12 h?), 21 events (1.1%) in the 12–24 h group, and nine events (1.1%) in the 24–48 h group. A multivariate regression analysis revealed that cardioversion after 12 h of symptom onset increased the risk of embolic complications more than threefold. The small number of events led to wide confidence intervals, but the p values reached statistical significance.
- Age (odds ratio [OR]: 1.05; 95% CI: 1.02–1.08), female sex (OR: 2.1; 95% CI: 1.1–4.0), heart failure (OR: 2.9; 95% CI: 1.1–7.2), and diabetes (OR: 2.3; 95% CI: 1.1–4.9) were the independent predictors of definite embolic events.

Classification tree analysis showed that the highest risk of thromboembolism (9.8%) was observed among patients with heart failure and diabetes, whereas patients with no heart failure and age < 60 years had the lowest risk of thromboembolism (0.2%).

Cardioversion with Corvert to prevent shock-induced sudden muscular contraction which may dislodge the implanted prosthesis. Our example patient "Jo Lar" was thus converted to "Low Risk Patient":

Cardio-orthopedics: specific treatment protocols to treat the heart without injuring the TJA

- Surgery: L hip replaced
- Post-op atrial flutter/atrial fibrillation—start Corvert within 12 h then antiarrhythmic meds or if >12 h TEE/CV → NSR.
- or
- Pre-op rhythm recording → Atrial Flutter/Fibrillation episodes, treat with perioperative antiarrhythmic meds.

7.3 Case 2 Report

Patient is a 79-year-old single female for R THA. She has been very active until recently because of her hip. She has had a L TKA in the past associated with the complication of pulmonary emboli. She has hypertension controlled with losartan 50 mg and hydrochlorothiazide 25 mg with no evidence of left ventricular hypertrophy on her echocardiogram or ECG. She has first degree AV block. Her echocardiogram shows a normal ejection fraction of 70% and a speckle tracking strain of 23.2%. Her carotid ultrasound and abdominal aorta ultrasound were normal.

Would this patient be considered a high risk patient? Her coronary CCTA showed a significant area of narrowing in the mid-LAD after the second diagonal vessel. There was a 76% narrowing with a lipid lake that constituted the plaque necrotic core which was not concentrated but was disorganized and not confluent. There was a plaque convergent—divergent double cone. The first diagonal vessel shows a narrowing at its origin of 39% with insignificant liquid lake. The circumflex and right coronaries showed no severe disease although the vessels showed artifact that had to be read around and made the images ineligible for HeartFlow analysis for coronary blood flow. The speckle tracking strain is normal at 23.2% with abnormal being—14% or greater.

The patient LAD plaque dashboard shows readily by illustration that the mid-LAD has a red zone which means danger alert. There is no ulcerated plaque but there are necrotic cores, 76% stenosis, and convergent-divergent double cones.

We studied this lesion comprehensively and decided to lower the risk by coding yellow as a warning and that this lesion in our experience would not be a high risk for a major adverse cardiac event (MACE).

Charlson Score 3 for age 79, all else 77% 10-year Survival:

- RCRI Score 0.
- Canadian score 0, but risk of LDL unknown.
- Reducible OSCARs 5 from CCTA 3, PE/DVT 2 -, high risk. - > reduced to 2 after deciding that coronary lesions without ulcer is low risk.
- ASA 1, severe systemic disease excluded, CAD with stent excluded, ischemia excluded by 85% echo negative speckle tracking.

Another score that is actively used is the Charlson Score named after Mary Charlson, an epidemiologist and department leader at Cornell Weil Medical School [4]. This was first developed by Dr. Carlson et al. in 1987 to predict death within a year of hospitalization. This score is frequently used in orthopedics although designed now for prediction of 10-year survival of patients with multiple comorbidities. The 18 current assessments are age, myocardial infarction, CHF, PAD, CVA or TIA, dementia, COPD, connective tissue disease, PUD, liver disease, DM, hemiplegia, CKD, solid tumor, leukemia, lymphoma, AIDS, and COVID-19. The Carlson Score is zero.

The modified Goldman risk score is only E. Age > 70. That would be two or fewer E-H which means this is low risk.

Total RCRI points 0.

ASA PS 1 normal Healthy patients.

OSCARs: CAD 3 + Hx of Pulmonary Embolus + 2 = 5. But with no plaque ulcers, CAD-RADs score [5] is in my experience in an asymptomatic patient having what has been classified as intermediate risk surgery, is of little risk which is why we are not proceeding to coronary intervention. Since we have weighted OSCARs to be reducible (Fig. 7.3), I will revise the score by calling CAD zero and still factor in the history of pulmonary emboli, that is 2, whereby risk is only moderate. The plan is to use guideline-based post-op enoxaparin for patients with a prior history of pulmonary emboli.

Possible Weighted Scores for Rescoring

OSCARs

RISK CLASS	POINTS
Low Risk	0 , 1
Moderate Risk	2 , 3
Severe Risk	4 or greater

Fig. 7.3 This is the score that we use for OSCAR; Low score is 0–1, moderate score is 2–3, and severe risk is 4 or greater; when a risk factor does not require intervention with a stent or if it is treatable and can be controlled medically, we down grade the risk by lowering the reducible OSCAR score (not reproduced)

Risk and plan: Lovenox (40 mg SQ q 24 h for 30 days) with a nurse navigator.

Patient had successful TJA surgery, no evidence of a cardiac event or symptoms, and treated with enoxaparin without developing pulmonary emboli. After 2 years follow-up, she has remained well and very active with her dancing.

A very nice article was written in 2019 with Dr. KAUSHIK HAZRATWALA as an orthopedist author and Yassin Elsiwy, a surgical resident [6]. They reviewed the literature including 15 studies in their data base and concluded at the end that "ultimately this data can be used in the development of an extensive preoperative risk assessment tool that can guide cardiology intervention to minimize cardiac complication post-THA and TKA." We perceived this as a challenge to our team.

Then Elsiwy group followed with a very nice retrospective article [7], looking at the risk factors of a group 274 of their patients seen from 2010 until end of 2017 who were asymptomatic and reviewed how they were treated by the seven cardiologists involved in their care and the sole orthopedist. All patients had ECGs and echoes which is normal in Queensland but not common elsewhere; in some of our bundled patients evaluated by other cardiologists and operated upon by other orthopedists, it was common to get an ECG 27/27 (100%) but rare to get an echo 2/27 (7%).

The Elsiwy et al. patients were found to have risk factors of increasing age, history of CVAs, FH of CAD, or discovered LV dysfunction by echo which were predictive of cardiovascular disease with 50 patients requiring additional testing which found: 1 with valvular heart disease, 2 with significant stenosis on CCTA, 12 with atrial fibrillation or heart block and 15 with abnormal coronary angiograms making a total of 17 (17/274 = 6%) in the CAD category. How the patients with coronary artery disease were treated either medically or with intervention was never mentioned as well as to whether they ever had TJR? Postoperative arrhythmia of atrial fibrillation was present in seven patients giving total PAF 19 total (19/274 = 6.9%). These results were encouraging to our group to accept the Elsiwy challenge by our development of a prospective study of 430 TJA patients with testing of ECG, echo, and adding ICA and Abdominal Aorta U/S, and CCTA to use in the develop of the OSCARs: Orthopedic Surgery Cardiovascular Anatomy Risk score for the assessment of inpatient/outpatient morbidity risk/medical Rx/stent. Given the fact that the asymptomatic group had a history of discovery of cardiovascular disease it seemed reasonable to assess all patient with anatomical data to discover their risk. Likewise it seemed reasonable to look 30 days before surgery so as to have significant time to treat the findings medically before surgery. We also determined that all prior risk scores were fixed and could not be reduced with treatment but that it might be valuable to have a risk that was reducible by recognition and treatment which we began to do as part of our study.

The Waterman Study also looked at risk analysis. They looked at increased risk of increasing length of stay and concluded that this increases with THA, age > 75 or 80, cardiovascular comorbidities, renal disease, and increasing risk scores ASA 3 severe or 4 severe and constant but does not include 5, which refers to moribund [8].

They concluded that their risk score was superior to the RCRI in predicting cardiovascular events from TJA.

In the Crash-Joint study [9], consisting of 65 patients for THA and 25 patients for TKA, showed cardiovascular risk factors with higher prevalence than the general population.

This is a good point to review the development of risk assessment historically and how that this has been used and whether it has been useful in orthopedics. When I wrote my chapter in 1983 called "Invasive Testing" Noncardiac Surgery in the Cardiac Patient," edited by Stephen P. Glasser Futura Publishing Company 1983 [10], I was using the Modified Goldman Risk Factors revised from 1977 for perioperative morbidity [11]. This had been proceeded by the simple Goldman Risk Score. This modified Goldman Risk was centered around recent MI in the last 6 months, arrhythmias, and aortic stenosis as 3 of the 4 cardiac risk factors which did not appear to be relevant as cardiology progressed from recent MI, aortic stenosis, and Holter monitor to less MI and AS in patients now assessed by echocardiography as a readily available and frequently available resource and as the approach to preoperative evaluation became multifactor which led to the Lee-Goldman RCRI. This original RCRI was then replaced by the Revised Cardiac Risk Index with update of content [12]. The score is 0 or 1 for six simple questions about elevated-risk surgery, history of ischemic heart disease, history of congestive heart failure, history of cerebral vascular disease, treatment with insulin, and preoperative elevated creatinine leading to a cumulative summation score. This tabulation gives 4 classes I–IV going from Class I 0.4% 30 day, Class II 0.9%, Class III 6.6%, to a final Class IV > 11% 30 day risk of death, MI, or cardiac arrest. Obviously, this score is designed to predict life-threatening events based on mostly three historical events, risky surgery, or IDDM or kidney failure which can miss many of the specific problems of lessor significance which can result in readmission in a bundled patient but is not a threat of death such as obesity, hypertension out of control, PAF, or an NSTEMI. These problems are to be avoided to escape bundled CMS penalties associated with prolonged admission, readmission, or disruption of outpatient surgery.

The OSCAR score is based on anatomical data from the echocardiogram, ultrasound of the abdominal aorta and carotid arteries, and computed coronary tomographic arteriogram. Treatment gives an opportunity to reduce the risk going into surgery for TJA. We think that this scoring is a change in physicians' patterns and recommend keeping a checklist so as not to err [13]. In our study of 430 patients for TJA, we did neglect to treat one patient with LVH and newly diagnosed HTN who came out of TJA with an elevated BP and congestive heart failure necessitating an extra day in the hospital. These are the structural anatomical biomarkers that we monitor in our patients 30 days before TJA to calculate the OSCARs which can be reduced by treatment:

- Hypertensive crisis, LVH
- PAF
- LAE
- Stroke
- Heart attack damage, CAD, plaque with diameter narrowing and plaque ulcer
- Abdominal aortic aneurysm leading to rupture risk
- Hypotension from aortic stenosis > no regional block

What we learned

3 Main Points to take away:

1) Cardiovascular Disease is the leading cause of complications in those > 65 y/o for elective hip or knee!

2) Cardiac risk "reducible" OSCARs is predictable, not random! Pieces of a puzzle: AS Gen anesth or not regional, TAA/AAA, HTN/LVH >12, 24 hr BP /CHF, PAF/TIA/CVA, PE/DVT, CAD/MACE/Platelets + Plaque ulcer , low EF and can be treated , "Reducible" =/means response reduced risk

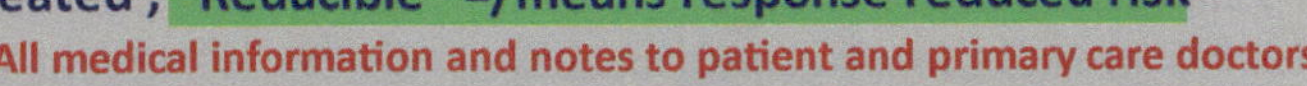

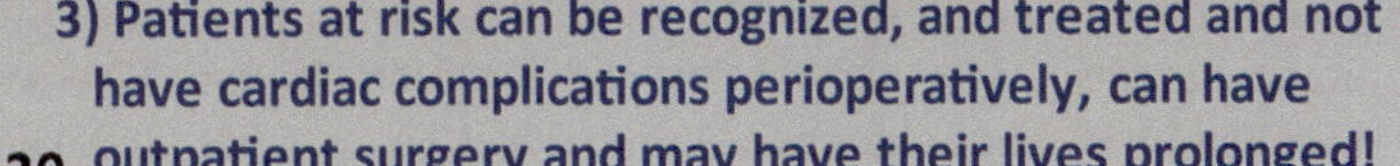

14-20

If you had three points to carry away acquired in this book without complications, these would be the most valuable card you could carry in your pocket. It makes a point of the most risky non-orthopedic complications, recognizes **OSCARs (Orthopaedic Surgery Cardiovascular Anatomical Risk** score) and the pieces of the puzzle currently recognized by identification of the current pieces of the puzzle. Our treatment protocols can lesson risk, and the possibility of TJA cannot be complicated by cardiovascular problems and the possibilities that this recognition and the management of cardiovascular risk my prolong life!

7.4 Case Report

JW is a bright energetic 86-year-old female who has spent her married and widowed life on a very busy farm in North Tampa. She has known coronary artery disease with stents over the years and later main left CAD treated with CABG with good results and still normal LV function on echoes. In a prep for surgery in 30 days, she was found to have a normal thoracic aorta but a dilated abdominal aorta by ultrasound of the abdomen, part of our routine evaluation for upcoming TKA. Because of her active life she wanted us to look closely with abdominal aortography which showed a fusiform saccular sub-renal arterial 5.2 cm aneurysm with a 5% chance of rupture (see Slide 1). The patient elected repair which was done with a Medtronic Endurant graft system. She only lost 100 cc of blood had a quick recovery and had a normal TKA without problems and at her scheduled time which was 13 days after aortic endograft.

I have had a lot of experience with aortic aneurysms and in fact know the patient's concern when she needs a knee and remembers her father having TKA successfully only to rupture an unknown abdominal aortic aneurysm and die 3 days later. This is uncommon and we have the means to detect it on our preoperative screening.

The presence of hypertension in 75% of our patients may make this more common. Those who have LVH without having had a diagnosis of hypertension until we saw them would be included.

Of our group of patients, five had moderate aortic stenosis without dilated aortas or RA, in which we recognized that they would have abnormal tilt table test-induced hypotension by past studies in AS patients and avoid in our patient regional anesthesia where this will be seen and therefore use general anesthesia.

Of 3 patients with more than mild AR, all female, 2 were moderate, and 1 was severe. One of the moderates had TAA of 48 mm. None had known RA.

Thirty-four had aortic dilatation of which 4, 2M and 2F, were abdominal only with our case patient having stenting of the 52 mm AAA, the only one meeting AA criteria. One male had both thoracic (42) and abdominal (40) with HTN and LVH. Of the 19 males (65%) with thoracic aortic dilatation, 16 were 39–44 mm and 3 were 45–48 mm. Fifteen of the 19 had HTN and 12 with LVH. Of the 10 females (35%) with dilated thoracic aortas, 7 were 38–42 mm and 3 had 45–48 mm. Five of the females had HTN and LVH. Thus among the group 6 had TAAs, 3 Ms (16%) and 3 Fs (30%) none of which required surgery yet.

7.5 Pulmonary Emboli and DVT

Cardio-orthopedists encounter a lot of patients who have a history of DVTs and DVT with pulmonary emboli. The problem existed in the past with such frequency that the AAOS has 183 pages of guidelines for prevention. Commonly at this point, an aspirin dose is commonly started postoperatively for prophylaxis. The use of ASA is no differently statistically from rivaroxaban or low molecular weight heparin. Many have a history of DVT or PE when they had surgery in the past, frequently TJA. Some have had resolution and are still on the medication they were treated with when diagnosed. These will stop their direct oral anticoagulants (DOACs) prior to surgery as instructed in the package insert for the standard drug and resume the drug when the surgeon is satisfied that the patient will not bleed from the surgical incision. Patients who had prior DVT or PE and had completed their 6 months of treatment will be started on the protocols recommended traditionally: If DVT then low molecular weight heparin 30 mg q 12 h for 14 days or if PE low molecular weight heparin q 24 h for 30 days.

Of the 430 cardio-orthopedics patients, there are 21 documented cases of patients with current or prior DVTs. Of the 21 documented cases of patients with current or prior DVTs, 10 patients also had documented PEs, either prior or currently.

Of the 430 cardo-orthopedics patients, there are 14 documented cases of patients with current or prior PEs. Of the 14 documented cases of patients with PEs, 10 had documented DVTs and 4 did not have documented DVTs.

There were three patients with new acute PEs who were asymptomatic who had TJA cancelled, were treated medically, and then went to surgery without problems.

We routinely do coagulopathy workups on patients who have TIA, CVAs, PEs, or DVTs looking for an etiology. Also preoperative patients get a laboratory workup frequently consisting of a complete blood count with PT and sometimes with PTT. Sometimes we bump into abnormal laboratory testing such as the following on a 53-year-old WM with PTT 38.2, APTT 40, repeat APPT 51.1, DRVVT 51.6, and cardio IGM > 112. Another repeat PTT was 30, dilute PT 51, dpt conf ratio 1.07, and dRVVT mix 39.9 were normal. The others are all only slightly abnormal. AD Beta 2 Glyco IGG, IGA, and IGM were normal. We reviewed all of these studies with our pathologist.

As you see review of the PT and PTT sometimes shows abnormal elevations. We then take a careful history of historical evidence of thrombocytosis which can be negative. Our workup then consists of APPT, PTT, lupis anticoagulant level DRVVT, anticardiolipin A with cardio IGG, IGA, and IGM, antiB2 glycoprotein antibody. Even though these are slightly elevated, risk in orthopedic surgery is no different from other orthopedic cases if there is no past history of thrombosis.

Note patients on lenalidomide with multiple myeloma are at high risk of blood clots and dexamethasone adds to that risk. Since it is given on days 0–21 and interrupted 22–28, we recommend the TJA during the pause period with oncology guidance as to when to restart (pt 58).

7.6 Risk Factor Pearls

There are many factors seen in this complex group of patients that are considered incidentalomas that are rarer but still important to cover. They are as follows:

- There were also patients with elevated serum creatinine seen as Stage III kidney disease that would be from excessive NSAIDs exposure. It was recommended that these patients stop the NSAIDS, check blood pressure and don't get dehydrated during surgery.
- Surgery is delayed for chronic severe anemia to find out if it is true, new, and treatment. NSAID-induced gastric bleeding is common.
- CT nodules discovered during CCTA are investigated prior to surgery. AI-assisted interpretation is helpful.
- Q waves are common in the inferior leads and will be ruled out as inferior wall infarctions by normal echo and CCTA wall motion as well as normal coronaries.
- Some patients have a history of hypotension and need to be well hydrated and perhaps an antihypertensive drug withheld.
- Patients with newly installed stents need to follow the anti-platelet company and interventionist recommendation as to when the drugs may be withheld for surgery and the risk of interruption. More chronic stent therapy can be withheld for surgery again as recommended.
- Patients with CABG with some occluded grafts need to have the reason for the graft occlusions which may be because of minimal or mild native vessel lesions which are not significantly occluded to sustain grafts. Or if the grafts go to infarctions which will not represent potential ischemic areas.

- Patients with borderline or severe LVH need to have BP 24 h monitoring to establish the diagnosis of HTN or sleep studies to eliminate ASO. LVH is the most frequent cause of PAF which will need several days to a week of Zio monitoring to be eliminated as a risk factor.
- Doctors to be alert of nickel and other mineral allergies usually represented as dermatological lesions.
- Mild and moderate AS patients need general rather than regional anesthesia with adequate hydration.
- Patients on coumadin for antithrombotic therapy with have 10% requiring very low dose and 10% requiring very high dose. Beware of this when restarting coumadin after having stopped it.
- All allergies need to specially noted and highlighted for anesthesia.
- Hypothyroidism is common and needs to be rechecked with TSF.
- COPD patients need to be given their inhalers.
- ASO patients as inpatients need to bring their CPAP.
- Patients having previous anthracycline should have strain echo to check for less than -14%.
- Patients with L breast radiation therapy need to be on the cardiac track for echo for LV function.
- Patients with III CKD should have spironolactone held.
- Pacemakers and ICDs do not need to have a magnet applied because of hip or knee distance from the pacer box unless it is implanted in a non-upper thoracic site.
- Patients with IVC filters that have been in continuous implantation will still need anticoagulation.
- Patients with significant stenosis in a single or two vessels on CCTA with reduced flow but no ulcers should be navigated by a nurse navigator.
- Carotid plaque calcification and stenosis with ipsilateral active cerebral symptoms is rare but should be investigated.
- High calcium score with heavy calcification can be sent to HeartFlow for analysis of coronary flow. Please note the 15% false positive with a 95% decreased flow and a 50% false positive with a 75% decreased flow by HeartFlow.
- Patients with Addison's disease should have perioperative increase in steroid dose by the endocrinologist.
- Previous history of AF ablation must be assessed by Continuous Heart Rhythm monitoring (> 24 hrs) for breakthrough PAF which occurs at the rate of 5% per year.
- CLL untreated is not considered increased risk.
- Past history of cardiac cath in the last year replaces the need for a new CCTA unless there are new stents or CABGs.
- Hypertension without LVH implies adequate BP medical treatment but with severe LVH means undertreatment with meds or also OSA. Frequently, antihypertensive drugs are continued on the day of surgery with sips of water.
- Patients with low EF < 35% need to be on aggressive medical management. They will do fine with mild NT-Pro BNP elevation.

- Very complicated cardiac patients with MVR, multiple stents, and aggressive medical management do well.
- Patients with mild elevation of Trop and BNP with TYPE II MI do well on medical Rx.
- General anesthesia is preferred to regional in Parkinson's disease patients because of hypotension.
- Patients with ECGs showing frequent PACs or a history of palpitations should have a Continuous Heart Rhythm monitoring (> 24 hrs) for several days to exclude PAF.
- Elevated RVSP above 50 mmHg indicates severe MR, COPD, or PEs.
- Your anesthesia preference and the reason should be listed.
- History of HCOM can result in significant SOB. Control with medications is indicate. Mevacanten is to be approved by the FDA soon. Check for PAF by Continuous Heart Rhythm monitoring (> 24 hrs).
- Patients sometimes decline our requested CCTA, Continuous Heart Rhythm monitoring (> 24 hrs), or echo for personal reasons or if they are under the care of stress test doctors or binary decision stent doctors. You can get by this obstacle by saying that you have been cared far to prevent ordinary events in everyday life, but this is an extraordinary event because of the release of bone powder and its activating platelets which can be harmful under certain circumstances. If doctors question you, you can answer by we are doing research and have created a registry.
- Seeing patients 30 days before surgery gives you the time for treatment and lowering thc OSCARS!
- Rheumatoid arthritis patients require special attention because of the use of disease modifying antirheumatic drugs (DMARDs). These consists of conventional DMARDs, biologic DMARDs, and targeted synthetic DMARDs. One of these, tofacitinib, in higher doses can cause blood clots.
- Psoriatic arthritis has been shown by Caristo investigators to increase inflammation of the coronary arteries such that fat attenuation goes up and can be treated with inflammation reducing drugs which will lower the coronary inflammatory risks.
- Sympathomimetics and catecholamines need to be avoided in patients with carcinoid disease but vasopressin and octreotide may be used. Patients take Sandostatin injection monthly which maybe stepped up prior to surgery.
- Eliquis 2.5 mg bid for 15 days may be used postoperatively in those with a prior history of DVT.
- Patients with moderate obstructive disease and a plaque ulcer can be navigating by an RN but have not had a significant problem postoperatively,
- To hold eliquis, withhold four doses before surgery. Hold Xarelto for three doses/48 h. Restart when ok with ortho.
- Mid LAD stenosis of 37% with a drop in HeartFlow 97% to 88% to 67% is not a serious change and may have surgery. Patient with 59% diameter lesion in the lad after the D1 with HeartFlow 94–78% had surgery without problems (NCS 26%, NCP 18%).

- Some patients with CAF and TVR will require an enoxaparin bridge when coumadin is stopped.
- Rare patients are denied CCTA by insurance age < 65.
- Patients frequently have history of vasovagal episodes during regional anesthesia but not during general.
- Chronic AF is not the same risk for CVA/TIA as PAF.
- Some patients have drug-induced atrial arrhythmias which may be resolved suggest telemetry post-op.

References

1. Mont MA, Jacobs JJ, Boggio LN, et al. Preventing venous thromboembolic disease in patients undergoing elective hip and knee arthroplasty. J Am Acad Orthop Surg. 2011;19(12):768–76.
2. Fleisher LA, Beckman JA, Brown KA, et al. ACC/AHA 2007 guidelines on perioperative cardiovascular evaluation and care for noncardiac surgery: a report of the American College of Cardiology/American Heart Association task force on practice guidelines (writing committee to revise the 2002 guidelines on perioperative cardiovascular evaluation for noncardiac surgery): developed in collaboration with the American Society of Echocardiography, American Society of Nuclear Cardiology, Heart Rhythm Society, Society of Cardiovascular Anesthesiologists, Society for Cardiovascular Angiography and Interventions, Society for Vascular Medicine and Biology, and Society for Vascular Surgery. Circulation. 2007;116(17):e418–99.
3. Tabatabaee RM, Rasouli MR, Rezapoor M, et al. Coronary revascularization and adverse events in joint arthroplasty. J Surg Res. 2015;198(1):135–42.
4. Charlson ME, Pompei P, Ales KL, MacKenzie CR. A new method of classifying prognostic comorbidity in longitudinal studies: development and validation. J Chronic Dis. 1987;40(5):373–83.
5. Cury RC, Abbara S, Achenbach S, et al. CAD-RADSTM Coronary Artery Disease e Reporting and Data System. An expert consensus document of the Society of Cardiovascular Computed Tomography (SCCT), the American College of Radiology (ACR) and the North American Society for Cardiovascular Imaging (NASCI). Endorsed by the American College of Cardiology. J Am Coll Radiol. 2016;13(12 Pt A):1458–1466.e9.
6. Elsiwy Y, Jovanovic I, Doma K, et al. Risk factors associated with cardiac complication after total joint arthroplasty of the hip and knee: a systematic review. J Orthop Surg Res. 2019;14(1):15.
7. Elsiwy Y, Symonds T, Doma K, et al. Pre-operative clinical predictors for cardiology referral prior to total joint arthroplasty: the 'asymptomatic' patient. J Orthop Surg Res. 2020;15(1):513.
8. Waterman BR, Belmont PJ Jr, Bader JO, Schoenfeld AL. The Total joint arthroplasty cardiac risk for predicting perioperative myocardial infarction and cardiac arrest after primary Total knee and hip arthroplasty. J Arthroplast. 2016;31(6):1170–4.
9. Łęgosz P, Kotkowski M, Platek AE, et al. Assessment of cardiovascular risk in patients undergoing total joint alloplasty: the CRASH-JOINT study. Kardiol Pol. 2017;75(3):213–20.
10. Harrison EE. Invasive testing. In: Glaser SP, editor. Noncardiac surgery in the cardiac patient: assessment and management. Austin: Futura Publishing Co; 1983.
11. Goldman L, Caldera DL, Nussbaum SR, et al. Multifactorial index of cardiac risk in noncardiac surgical procedures. N Engl J Med. 1977;297(16):845–50.
12. Lee TH, Marcantonio ER, Mangione CM, et al. Derivation and prospective validation of a simple index for prediction of cardiac risk of major noncardiac surgery. Circulation. 1999;100(10):1043–9.
13. Gawande A, editor. The checklist manifesto: how to get things right, vol. 1. 1st ed. NY: Metropolitan books, Henry Holt and Co; 2000. p. 64.

Hypertension

8

Eric E. Harrison

Abstract

This chapter introduces by way of case review, anecdotal evidence and evidence-based experience, the need for closer cooperation between orthopedics and cardiology, particularly in relation to total joint arthroplasty (TJA). Hypertension, combined with LVH, increases cardiovascular risk. Numerous ramifications of hypertension in multiorgan damage, such as the development of dementia or cognitive decline, renal artery stenosis and progressive renal disease, and certainly the addition of coronary artery disease in the long term, which are not to be taken lightly and certainly cannot be ignored in the interval follow-up with echocardiograms.

Keywords

Left ventricular hypertrophy (LVH) · Echocardiogram (Echo) · Renal artery stenosis · Total joint arthroplasty (TJA) · Coronary artery disease (CAD) Hypertension (HTN)

8.1 Case Presentation 1

EL is a 79-year-old female for R THA. she has LVH of 13 mm, EF 68%, moderate calcific carotid plaque. CAR-RADs 1 and no PAF by Continuous Heart Rhythm Monitoring (> 24 hrs) and normal ECG. There is a history of GERD. Creatinine is

E. E. Harrison (✉)
Board Chair International Cardio-Oncology Society, ICOS CEO PrivaCors Inc. Cardio-Orthopaedics®, Tampa, FL, USA

Department of Medicine, Morsani College of Medicine, University of South Florida, Tampa, FL, USA

Joint Special Operations University, MacDill Air Force Base, Tampa, FL, USA

E. E. Harrison, N. H. Ho (eds.), *Managing Cardiovascular Risk In Elective Total Joint Arthroplasty*, https://doi.org/10.1007/978-3-031-26415-3_8

0.6. She was begun on Edarbidchlor 40/12.5 and her recorded BPs came down some but adding amlodipine 5 mg per day normalized it. She had TJA without problems.

8.2 Case Presentation 2

PD is a 77-year-old female for outpatient L TKA. She denies any history of hypertension, diabetes, or CAD. She has a history of elevated cholesterol. ECG shows an NSR with NSSTTW changes. Echo shows LVH of 13 mm, EF 76%, less than 50% carotid plaque, and Continuous Heart Rhythm Monitoring (> 24 hrs) negative for PAF after 2 days. Her CAD-RADs is 3 with a less than 70% Ca plaque without obstruction. She is sensitive to tape and has a PCN allergy. Her blood pressure was 160/85. She was not treated with new anti-hypertensive medications by an oversight. This was before we developed our OSCARS checklist modeled after that of Atul Gawande in the "Checklist Manfesto" so that treatment would not fall through the cracks [1]. After surgery, her BP was markedly elevated and she developed CHF with SOB. She was admitted to the hospital and treated with anti-hypertensive medications and a diuretic, CHF, and BP elevation resolved and she was discharged home.

This patient had LVH 13 with undiagnosed hypertension but was not started on medications by our error. After TKA, she developed CHF and uncontrolled hypertension for which she was admitted and received aggressive treatment and was controlled and discharged the following day. This shows the importance of having a checklist so in using OSCARs no patient goes untreated. Frequently, we gave the anti-hypertensive medications the day of surgery with sips of water. We have not noted adverse effects operatively or postoperatively.

In the CRASH-JOINT Study, 55.6% of patients (n = 50) were diagnosed with HTN based on past history [2]. They also recorded 24-h blood pressure surveillance. In this group with abnormal ambulatory BP recordings, 45.6% of patients were consistent with hypertension. Echocardiogram diagnosis of LVH was not mentioned. This implies inadequate treatment. Atrial fibrillation was not noted. 24.6% were smokers. Overall, early diagnosis and treatment was recommended. Łęgosz and his group also introduced the term "cardio-orthopedics" [3].

Elsiwy, et al. showed that the most common risk was hypertension at 65.2%. Echo cardiograms were routinely performed, but there was no mention of LVH having been found in patients with or without hypertension [4].

In "Risk factors associated with cardiac complication after total joint arthroplasty of the hip and knee: a systematic review," his group showed that hypertension in some quoted studies was related to cardiovascular complications and in others was not [5].

The number of people aged 30–79 living with hypertension has doubled to 1.28 billion since 1990 with more than 700 million people with untreated hypertension! World Health Organization (WHO) and Imperial College London, Joint News Release, August 25, 2021.53% of women and 62% of men were not having BP control with only ¼ women and 1/5 men having adequate control. In addition, 41% of women and 51% of men were unaware they had hypertension. As far as hypertension treatment, this amounts to 73% of all women with hypertension and 66% of all men with hypertension in the USA. New "Guidelines for the Pharmacological treatment of hypertension in adults" have been developed by the WHO in 2021 [6].

In our Study of 430 patients for elective TJA over the age of 65 year old, hypertension occurred in 75%,and LVH occurred in 50%, due to more HTN or OSA or both. Echocardiography was of great aid in discovering these covert diseases and beginning treatment with hopefully 30 days to see the patient once a week to titrate medications to BP control. 24 h BP recordings were useful for deciding about control. Sleep studies were necessary to discover whether OSA was a contributor to elevated BP, LVH, or PAF. The LVH was a frequent marker for occult PAF, thus requiring Continuous Heart Rhythm Monitoring (> 24 hrs).

Hypertension combined with LVH increases cardiovascular risk and shows long-term undertreatment of hypertension [7]. Adequate treatment with BP control can resolve HTN and reverses LVH. This would signify significant blood pressure control. There are numerous ramifications of hypertension in multiorgan damage such as the development of dementia or cognitive decline, renal artery stenosis, and progressive renal disease, and certainly the addition of coronary artery disease in the long term which are not to be taken lightly and certainly cannot be ignored by not seeing the patients in interval follow-up with echocardiograms instead of not rescheduling them because they are asymptomatic from silent hypertension, a proposal some times endorsed my national health systems to make available more slots for clinical evaluation of those who are symptomatic.

Common frequent causes of hypertension are smoking, being overweight or obese, lack of physical activity, too much salt in the diet, too much alcohol consumption (more than 1–2 drinks per day), stress, older age, and genetics.

Patients who are candidates for TJA not surprisingly have sometimes up to 6 years of progressive osteoarthropathy with stages of treatment with PT, steroid injection, stem cell injection, NSAID use, continued aging, weight gain, prolonged inflammatory reactions, hypertension with TVH, metabolic syndrome, loss of activation of 500 genes because of exertional inactivity that in totality results in a decline in overall healthiness. The guidelines seem to be set at a point of almost total inactivity before a surgical solution is activated. This may result in some non-reversible changes that would indicate prolonging activation of a surgical solution may be waiting too long and that earlier activation of TJA may result in better and quicker recovery. CMS may find better longevity with earlier surgical solutions. Orthopedists, as they review these chapters, need to reconsider the current guidelines in the light of the cardiovascular risks factor that we are showing.

References

1. Gawande A. The checklist manifesto: how to get things right. 1st ed. NY: Metropolitan books; 2000.
2. Łęgosz P, Kotkowski M, Platek AE, et al. Assessment of cardiovascular risk in patients undergoing total joint alloplasty: the CRASH-JOINT study. Kardiol Pol. 2017;75(3):213–20.

3. Łęgosz P, Płatek AE, Board TN, Szymański FM. Cardioorthopedics–is it necessary in clinical practice? A study of patients with hip replacement surgery. Kardiol Pol. 2017;75(8):729–35.
4. Elsiwy Y, Symonds T, Doma K, et al. Pre-operative clinical predictors for cardiology referral prior to total joint arthroplasty: the 'asymptomatic' patient. J Orthop Surg Res. 2020;15(1):513.
5. Elsiwy Y, Jovanovic I, Doma K, et al. Risk factors associated with cardiac complication after total joint arthroplasty of the hip and knee: a systematic review. J Orthop Surg Res. 2019;14(1):15.
6. WHO. Guideline for the pharmacological treatment of hypertension in adults. 2021. https://www.who.int/publications/i/item/9789240033986.
7. Lee HH, Lee H, Cho SMJ, et al. On-treatment blood pressure and cardiovascular outcomes in adults with hypertension and left ventricular hypertrophy. J Am Coll Cardiol. 2021;78(15):1485–95.

Troponins

9

Christopher J. Augustine and Eric E. Harrison

Abstract

This chapter introduces by way of case review, anecdotal evidence and evidence-based experience, the need for closer cooperation between orthopedics and cardiology, particularly in relation to total joint arthroplasty (TJA). To understand the use of fifth generation hs-tononin T in predicting cardiac events and its complexity in aiding predicting cardiac events in the nonoperative patient.

Keywords

Cardio orthopedics · Total joint arthroplasty (TJA) · Preoperative evaluation · Cardiac risk of TJA · Perioperative risk assessment · High sensitivity cardiac troponin T (hs-Troponin T) · VISION trial · Devereaux

To understand use of fifth-generation hs-troponin T in predicting cardiac events and the complexity of this, it is useful to examine the work of the experts in predicting cardiac events in the nonoperative patients first for heart attack prediction. A study by doctors Sandoval and Jaffe intended to optimize the use of the fifth-generation cardiac troponin T (hs-cTnT) assay for more rapid evaluations for myocardial

C. J. Augustine (✉)
International Society of Cardio-Orthopaedics, Tampa, FL, USA

E. E. Harrison
Board Chair International Cardio-Oncology Society, ICOS CEO PrivaCors Inc. Cardio-Orthopaedics®, Tampa, FL, USA

Department of Medicine, Morsani College of Medicine, University of South Florida, Tampa, FL, USA

Joint Special Operations University, MacDill Air Force Base, Tampa, FL, USA

E. E. Harrison, N. H. Ho (eds.), *Managing Cardiovascular Risk In Elective Total Joint Arthroplasty*, https://doi.org/10.1007/978-3-031-26415-3_9

infarction (MI), in addition to avoiding problems that are often associated with increased sensitivity testing [1]. Sandoval and Jaffe set out to guide clinicians' use of hs-cnTnT for acute cardiac care based on their evidence-based synopses. The authors define the hs-cTnT assay as an enzyme-linked immunosorbent assay with two monoclonal antibodies to amino acids 125–131 and 136–147 for the biotinylated, mouse-human chimera tag antibody. A difference between the fourth generation and the more sensitive fifth-generation assays are the values. Values for the fifth-generation hs-cTn assays are reported always as whole numbers. Thus, a fourth-generation value of 30 ng/mL in terms of the new fifth-generation hs-cTnT equates to 0.01 ng/mL. The "anchor values" to know for this adaptation are as follows: a value of 53 ng/mL equates to 0.03 mg/mL; a value of 100 ng/L equates to 0.1 ng/mL. The former three values are what constitutes these "anchor values." Together, they proposed that high sensitivity troponin assays should utilize sex-specific cut-offs, rule out myocardial infarction over 2 h in those who are below the 99th percentile upper reference limit, and strongly consider myocardial infarction in those who have values of >100 ng/L and/or a change >10 ng/L at 2 h.

The study also defines the limit of blank (LoB) and the limit of detection (LoD) which are analytic parameters used to describe the smallest concentrations of cTn measurable. They define the limit of quantitation (LoQ) as the lowest concentration that can be measured with a coefficient of variation <20%. Sandoval and Jaffe mention that these analytic parameters are the lowest limit that the FDA allows to be reported. They go on to outline the FDA LoB and LoD for hs-cTnT as 3 ng/mL and 5 ng/mL, respectively, for the cobas e 411 analyzer. For the cobas e 601 and cobas e 602 analyzer, the 2.5 mg/mL and 3 mg/mL, respectively, with an LoQ of 6 ng/mL for all.

A primary purpose of Sandoval and Jaffe's study was to advocate for ruling out values that are less than the 99th percentile upper reference limit and to use sex-specific cut-off of 10 ng/mL for women and 15 ng/mL for men. The authors refer to the clinical practice guidelines which endorse the use of the 99th percentile of cTn to support the diagnosis of acute myocardial injury and acute myocardial infarction. They go on to mention that in all studies, men have higher 99th percentiles than women and the authors endorse the values of 10 ng/mL for women and 15 ng/mL for men for hs-cTn assays.

Next, they discuss single-measurement strategies for ruling out myocardial infarction. In low-risk patients, Sandoval and Jaffe advocate for using the LoB and/or LoD in conjunction with a single hs-cTnT measurement at presentation with high sensitivity and a negative predictive value (NPV). The recent meta-analyses provided in the article shows that nearly one-third of the 9241 patient participants qualified for this type of assessment with a pooled sensitivity and an NPV of 98.7% (95% CI, 97.3–99.8). Sandoval and Jaffe maintain that this method should be used in patients who are low risk or present at least 2 h after the onset of symptoms due to data that expresses caution in early presenters. The reason they support this way of triage via hs-cTn is because this sensitive detection method of myocardial injury can also detect the comorbidities that lead to atherosclerosis since even the comorbidities cause increases in hs-cTnT within the normal range. Additionally, due to the imprecision at low levels as a result of the prior instrumentation, sensitivity of the assay, and FDA regulation, LoB or LoD cannot be used in the United States; however, Sandoval and Jaffe suspect that the use of the new fifth-generation single hs-cTn measurements below the LoD will be used to expedite the evaluation of low-risk patients.

The study also asserts that the rapid identification of patients at low risk using hs-cTnT seems plausible using serial measurements at hours 0, 1, and 2, after presentation. Sandoval and Jaffe are concerned about the 1-h rule that has been proposed by the European Society of Cardiology which stemmed from the change they made to the rule-out and rule-in criteria of <3 ng/mL and > 5 ng/mL, respectively. Sandoval and Jaffe maintain that the imprecision of the current assay format at low levels does indeed seem problematic for this ruling and, secondly, the European study had very few early presenters participating. As a result, the authors of this study do not agree with the 1-h rule-out strategy, and instead, support the 2-h rule-out protocol especially for low-risk patients.

The authors note that assessment of risk can be executed by the use of a validated clinical risk score and/or a 12-lead electrocardiogram (ECG). They mention a recent collaborative analysis that revealed: "normal ECG with serial measurements at 0/2 h <99th percentile with a Thrombolysis in Myocardial Infarction score ≤ 1 has a high sensitivity and NPV to exclude acute myocardial infarction and 30-day major adverse cardiac events." Furthermore, they recommend that clinicians integrate serial hs-cTnT measurements at 0/2 h at less than or equal to the sex-specific 99th percentile cut-offs in the absence of a change in values of 4 ng/L and combine that with a normal or nonischemic ECG and the patient's history or a validated risk score (preferred) to identify patients at low risk for early discharge. Sandoval and Jaffe identify a conservative protocol that would triage the patients who would need an additional third sample at the 4-h point. In high-risk patients, they identify them at various points along the 0- and 2-h mark, the requirements at the initial 0-h point is an hs-cTnT >100 ng/L which means they are at high risk for an acute MI and need prompt cardiac evaluation. However, if at their 2-h rule-out time their score is >1 hs-cTnT > sex-specific 99th percentiles, the patient is identified as having a myocardial injury and depending on if they have significant concentration change, can be triaged to the appropriate care for chronic myocardial injury or potential late MI, or acute MI or injury, or if necessary, prompt cardiac evaluation.

For ruling-in myocardial infarction, Sandoval and Jaffe first define the Universal Definition: an acute myocardial infarction is diagnosed when there is clinical evidence of acute myocardial ischemia and a rise and/or fall of cTn with at least one value greater than the sex-specific 99th percentile. Thus, the authors suggest that increases in hs-cTnT >99th percentile are consistent with myocardial injury but are not sufficient for a diagnosis of acute myocardial infarction. As a result, they bring up the numerous approaches that have been developed to facilitate the diagnosis of acute myocardial infarction for hs-cTn assays, such as the methods to use very high concentration (about five times the upper reference limit for hs-cTnT) and/or using the delta cTn to improve specificity of myocardial infarctions. They concede that these approaches do not adequately meet an ideal positive predictive value (PPV).

Sandoval and Jaffe maintain that these methods first need substantial improvement and modification before they can ever be implemented on a broader scale. They do, however, assert that the high-value approach can be functionally used to suggest acute myocardial infarction in patients with hs-cTnT concentrations >100 ng/L and for them to be considered for further cardiovascular evaluation. They uphold that altering change criteria (delta) further to distinguish smaller changes is problematic especially in patients who have low values because of the imprecision in detection. Furthermore, Sandoval and Jaffe advocate for the literature-supported absolute-criteria method (ng/L) as opposed to the percentage or relative criteria approach. Specifically, they support a conservative 10 ng/L change over a 2-h period to improve the diagnostic specificity for acute myocardial infarction.

Conversely, they also identify three more crucial aspects of ruling-in myocardial infarction. First of which, they advocate in patients who do not rule-out or rule-in for acute myocardial injury, as a result, they belong to the "intermediate zone" and require additional evaluation. These patients will need a third hs-cTnT value 2 h later and oftentimes will provide clarity in their diagnosis. They suggest criteria requiring a change of 12 ng/L in order to identify patients who are at higher risk of myocardial infarction. The second aspect they note is in patients who have presented late onset of symptoms (after 12 h). They believe that these patients should be considered to potentially be on the downslope of the time-concentration curve where it is difficult to observe the pattern-change in such a short amount of time. Thus, they urge responses to the slow or unchanging hs-cTnT values to not be concern-driven. Lastly, in patients who have values that are increasing at rates that are alarming but have not eclipsed the 99% URL threshold, Sandoval and Jaffe advise that these patients may be at substantial risk and require careful scrutiny and additional samples for further measurement of hs-cTnT. Alternatively, the same is true for patients who have increases that cause their values to surpass the 99th percentile range yet do not exceed the 10 ng/L.

In patients with elevated hs-cTnT values, Sandoval and Jaffe emphasize the primary importance of first assessing the pretest probability of atherothrombotic acute myocardial infarction before evaluating the hs-cTnT values. They offer an example comparing a patient in end-stage renal disease presenting with symptoms of dyspnea, a hs-cTnT value of 50 ng/L to a patient with the same values with typical angina and no confounding issues. Thus, marked increases (100 ng/L) on the initial sample indicate a higher risk and/or increased likelihood for acute myocardial infarction and immediate evaluation is necessary. In this instance, Sandoval and Jaffe recommend additional serial testing in order to best distinguish myocardial injury (e.g., from Sepsis) from myocardial infarction. The authors deemed it worth noting that despite the use of dynamic changes to determine myocardial infarction, dynamic changes also present in many other conditions such as acute pulmonary embolism, Takosubo cardiomyopathy, and myocarditis. Sandoval and Jaffe suggest that through the use of more high-sensitivity assays clinicians testing hs-cTnT levels in their patients will reveal problems that are not primarily cardiac-related, some being chronic and others being dynamic (e.g., sepsis). These patients are at increased risk due to their primary problem and must be triaged to a health care provider best-suited to treat that disease and not necessarily sent to a cardiology service. If hs-cTnT is high (>100 ng/L), Sandoval and Jaffe recommend cardiology consultation as well.

The researchers divulge that the fifth-generation hs-cTnT assay increases the frequency of acute myocardial infarction percentage compared to the less sensitive fourth-generation standard assay of 22–36%. Though, the incidence of acute myocardial infarction only modestly changes from 18–22% and in association with a reciprocal reduction in the incidence of unstable angina (13–11%). Sandoval and Jaffe declare that patients with newly diagnosed myocardial infarction represent a high-risk group of patients with increased mortality. Therefore, they believe, if the fifth-generation hs-cTnT assay is used appropriately, it should not lead to an increase in the use of coronary angiography.

Overall, this study resolves that using hs-cTnT assay will provide more sensitive and useful analytic data for clinicians and improve care. Sandoval and Jaffe reason that the identification of low-risk patients would be facilitated more rapidly, as well as the rule-in of acute myocardial injury. Likewise, if patients who potentially have acute myocardial ischemia also receive delta cTn measurements (or other metric tests), they can be better diagnosed and triaged for acute myocardial infarction and from there receive the appropriate interventions. Most importantly, they suggest that triaging patients using this approach is totally reliant upon the clinical context of the patients' primary diagnoses and not merely on isolated hs-cTnT values, even if increasing; patients with values >100 ng/L should receive a cardiac evaluation. Hopefully this will be utilized for TJA in the future with these careful considerations.

Through the breakdown and synopses of these three research studies, the usefulness of troponin tests in patients after surgery is clear. There are many different methods to conduct troponin tests, whether it be high sensitivity cardiac troponin T tests, using Cobas gen V, or pairing with delta cTn or NT-proBNP measurements in order to more accurately triage patients clinically and provide them with better care. In the sub-specialty of cardio-orthopedics, this assay would be utilized to better identify potential risks in patients post-operation.

The use of Troponin T assessment and measurement assays have recently been implemented more and more in clinical practices as a way to better assess patients' health risk post-surgery, and also as a marker for their general health. In the last few years, there have been several studies outlining the use of Troponin T or I assessment in patients' post-operation for a variety of clinical reasons. In this chapter, we will take a look into the pertinent research and explain why this information is so valuable to cardio-orthopedic cases. Our team set up Roche hs-Troponin T gen V Cobas platform testing for our research study in TJA over 65-year-old patients as preoperative evaluation only to find recurrent insurance denial of these tests [2]. We also had the same problem with NP-Pro-BNP and insurers. Therefore, this data will not be available for this group. That non-accumulation of chemical biomarkers warranted a thorough review of the existing literature to make up for the lack of data support in our research. We will explore the information available in general pre- and postoperative patients and hone I n on Cardio-orthopedics specifically when this data is available.

The prognostic effect of high-sensitive troponin T (hs-cTnT) assessment in elderly patients with chronic heart failure (HF) set out to analyze the value of hs-cTnT in patients with chronic heart failure as a predictor for further risk markers. Measurements for cardiac troponin T (cTnT) and troponin I (cTnI) have been previously introduced for the diagnosis of acute myocardial infarction (MI). However, analyzing troponin levels are not merely limited to predicting MI. As of late, predictions using hs-cTnT assessments are associated with diagnosis in patients with chronic heart failure (HF). Additionally, in these patients, the changes in cTnT monitored by hs-cTnT assay were revealed to predict cardiovascular events (CV). Although the hs-cTnT assay was able to further predict CV events, the discrimination of the type of CV was not anymore improved. The authors (Gravning et al) believe that the increase of HF incidence and prevalence in the growing elderly demographic warrants a deeper investigation into the role of elevated hs-cTnT in older patients with chronic HF. Thus, this more thorough exposition was done in 30% of the patients in the pre-existing CORONA trial called, which was performed on older patients with systolic HF of ischemic origin [3]. Rosuvastatin is a statin drug that is used for treating high cholesterol and triglyceride levels and can also be used to reduce the risk of MI, stroke, and other cardiac events. The CORONA trial found that rosuvastatin did not reduce the primary outcome of death from CV, fatal MI, nonfatal stroke, nor all-cause mortality. However, the evaluation of hs-cTnT in chronic HF, the CORONA trial assessed the predictive value of elevated baseline hs-cTnT and the predicted value changes in hs-cTnT from baseline to 3-month follow-up and further look into possible interactions with statin therapy. Gravning et al. hypothesized that hs-cTnT would provide additional prognostic and discriminating information beyond that of established HF risk factors in this patient cohort [4]. The methods for testing this hypothesis was from within the CORONA trial. The methods of the patient criteria are as follows: briefly, patients aged ≥60 years with chronic HF attributed to ischemic heart disease, defined as (1) medical history or ECG signs of old MI or (2) other data indication ischemic cause of HF (i.e., wall motion disturbances on echocardiography, left bundle branch block, or history of another occlusive atherosclerotic disease [i.e., earlier stroke, intermittent claudication, percutaneous coronary intervention]), who were in New York Heart Association (NYHA) class II–IV, with a left ventricular ejection fraction ≤40% (≤35% if NYHA II), were eligible, provided the investigator thought they did not need treatment with a cholesterol-lowering drug. The main criteria for exclusion were a recent CV event, current or planned procedures or operations, acute or chronic liver disease, serum creatinine ≥2.5 mg/dL, contraindications to statin therapy, or unexplained increase in creatine kinase. All patients provided written informed consent. Patients were randomly assigned to rosuvastatin 10 mg/d or matching placebo, once daily.

This study was a predefined substudy of the main CORONA trial and all patients provided written informed consent. Patients were randomly assigned to rosuvastatin 10 mg/day or a matching placebo, once daily. CORONA had 1480 patients and hs-cTnT was measured in 1245 of them, with samples available at both baseline and 3 months. The primary predefined outcome was the composite of death from CV causes, nonfatal MI, and nonfatal stroke analyzed as the time to the first event. Of secondary outcomes, the following were used in this substudy: (1) all-cause mortality, (2) CV mortality, and (3) composite of CV mortality and hospitalizations from worsening of HF (WHF). The definition and adjudication of all outcomes, as well as data on high-sensitivity C-reactive protein (hs-CRP) and amino-terminal pro-brain natriuretic peptide (NT-proBNP), have been described in detail.

The results of this study were that 1078 patients (86.6%) had hs-cTnT levels above the detection limit of 3 ng/L of the assay. Patients with hs-cTnT in the 99th percentile (14 ng/L) were separated into two groups: hs-cTnT levels >14 ng/L and hs-cTnT levels <14 ng/L. Patients with hs-cTnT levels >14 ng/L were found to be older, more often men, had lower left ventricular ejection fraction, lower body mass index, and higher heart rate than those with hs-cTnT levels <14 ng/L. Furthermore, patients with hs-cTnT levels >14 ng/L were found to have a higher prevalence of atrial fibrillation, other atherosclerotic diseases, previous percutaneous coronary intervention, diabetes mellitus, hypertension, and chronic obstructive pulmonary disease. Patients with hs-cTnT levels >14 ng/L were more commonly treated with aldosterone antagonists, diuretics, and digitalis glycosides. On the contrary, a history of angina pectoris and the use of β-blockers were less prevalent in patients hs-cTnT above the 99th percentile compared to those with hs-cTnT levels <14 ng/L. Patients with hs-cTnT levels >14 ng/L were also found to have lower total and low-density lipoprotein cholesterol levels and a lower average eGFR but had higher levels of NT-proBNP and hs-CRP. Next, the following variables were significantly associated with elevated hs-cTnT levels and were extrapolated into a linear regression model: NT-proBNP levels, diabetes mellitus, history of coronary revascularization, age, use of digitoxin/digoxin, diuretics and β-blockers, hs-CRP levels, systolic and diastolic blood pressures, heart rate, female sex, and eGFR remained independently associated with hs-cTnT levels, explaining 47.1% (R2) of the variation. Of these variables, NT-proBNP was the strongest predictor of elevated hs-cTnT levels. Moreover, there was no statistically significant interaction between hs-cTnT levels and treatment with rosuvastatin. The difference in hs-cTnT concentrations at baseline and 3-month follow-up were not statistically different, neither in the placebo group nor in the rosuvastatin group.

A median follow-up was done after 955 days, during which, it was found that 366 patients had died. Further analysis found linearity between risk for all-cause mortality and log-transformed hs-cTnT levels. Also, Kaplan-Meier plots for the primary endpoint, all-cause mortality, CV mortality, and the composite of CV mortality and hospitalization from worsening heart failure demonstrated a significantly higher frequency of events for patients with hs-cTnT levels >14 ng/L compared to those with hs-cTnT levels <14 ng/L. Importantly, hs-cTnT levels diverged according to the 99th percentile (14 ng/L) and remained a significant predictor of outcome in an extended multivariable regression model. Also, hs-cTnT levels were significant in predicting factors such as systolic and diastolic blood pressures, history of angina pectoris, history of atherosclerotic disease, history of previous revascularization, hypertension, atrial fibrillation, chronic obstructive pulmonary disease, total cholesterol, low-density lipoprotein levels, use of diuretics, use of aldosterone antagonists, use of β-blockers, and use of digitalis glycoside.

The addition of hs-cTnT in conjunction with hs-CRP and NT-proBNP variables significantly improved prognostic discrimination of the primary endpoint (cardiovascular death, nonfatal myocardial infarction, and nonfatal stroke), as well as all-cause mortality, CV mortality, and the composite of CV mortality and hospitalization from worsening heart failure (WHF).

All in all, the changes in hs-cTnT levels over time were as such: 300 patients (29%) had a >15% increase in hs-cTnT between baseline and 3 months. Of those patients, 183 (61%) had a baseline hs-cTnT <14 ng/L and 117 (39%) had a baseline hs-cTnT >14 ng/L. This increase was associated with a higher risk of composite endpoint of CV mortality or hospitalization because of worsening heart failure (WHF) but not with any of the other previously mentioned endpoints, including the primary endpoints of death from CV causes, nonfatal MI, and nonfatal stroke. Overall, elevated hs-cTnT levels in elderly patients with chronic HF of ischemic cause provide independent prognostic and discriminating information beyond that of established risk markers. The prognostic value of baseline hs-cTnT levels was superior to that of changes during follow-up.

The VISION study was conducted similarly in testing troponin levels by PJ Devereaux et al. a large international study that evaluated major complications after noncardiac surgery [5]. Participants had their troponin T (TnT) levels measured after noncardiac surgery, and the relationship between peak fourth-generation TnT level after noncardiac surgery and 30-day mortality were assessed. The eligible participants for the VISION study had noncardiac surgery were at least 45 years of age, received a general or regional anesthetic, and underwent elective, urgent, or emergency surgery. Patients had to consent to allow prognostic evaluation of fourth-generation TnT assay measurement, and the 24 potential preoperative predictors of 30-day mortality that were evaluated as well. Exclusion criteria were listed as patients who did not require an overnight hospital admission post-operation, if they declined consent, and if they were previously enrolled in the study.

Procedures for this study were as follows: Patients had blood collected and measured for a Roche fourth-generation Elecsys TnT assay 6–12 h postoperatively and on the first, second, and third days after surgery. Patients enrolled between 12 and 24 h after surgery had a TnT drawn immediately, and testing continued as previously described. Then the TnT measurements were analyzed at the contributing hospitals and reported to the attending physicians. The primary outcome was mortality at 30 days after surgery. This was monitored via phone call to each participant 30 days after surgery, and if the patient or the next of kin available informed that an occurrence of an outcome had happened, their physician was contacted and the study personnel received the proper documentation.

Regarding the analysis of the relationship between TnT levels and 30-day mortality, firstly, for the patients who did not answer the phone, the research personnel marked them according to the last day their health status was known. Furthermore, the percentage of patients who died within the range of 30 days after surgery and with a 95% confidence interval (CI). The researchers chose to use a Cox proportional hazards model to display this data and set the dependent variable as mortality up to 30 days after surgery, and the independent variables to include 24 preoperative factors. Then the same model was used with the addition of peak fourth-generation TnT measurement during the first 3 days post-surgery as an independent variable and a minimum *P*-value approach was used to determine if there were TnT threshold values that independently changed the patients' risk of mortality. This model approach was adapted to evaluate every possible threshold of TnT (e.g., <0.01, vs >0.01; <0.02 vs >0.02) in the Cox proportional model with the 24 preoperative factors.

Their analysis revealed that the TnT value that demonstrated the smallest statistically significant *P*-value was a TnT fixed threshold that independently predicted 30-day mortality. The Cox multivariable analysis was repeated until the research personnel could no longer identify any other statistically significant TnT thresholds. Additionally, the researchers used a Kruskal-Wallis test to determine if there were any significant differences in the median time from peak TnT value to death across the TnT threshold that was the independent predictor of 30-day mortality. For all independent predictors of 30-day mortality, the VISION study reported an adjusted hazard ratio (aHR), 95% CI, and associated *P*-value (a priori two-sided $a = 0.05$ was designated as statistically significant) through the method of bootstrapping 1000 samples. The VISION group used the Cox model to take into account any potential site-clustering, random-effects, and frailty and determined the likelihood ratios for the proportion of deaths that TnT threshold could possibly be responsible for. In their analysis, they classified 30-day mortality as low risk (<1%), intermediate risk (1–5%), high risk (>5–10%), and very high risk (>10%). The VISION group also analyzed whether there was a relationship between the preoperative estimated glomerular filtration rate and the TnT thresholds that independently predicted 30-day mortality in patients whom preoperative creatinine was measured. They set out to determine if the TnT thresholds in their model that included the peak TnT measurement continued to predict 30-day mortality, both vascularly and nonvascularly, based on the surgery center's determination of the cause of death.

The results of the VISION trial came from 15,133 eligible patients who received the fourth-generation TnT prognostic study, and 99.7% of them completed the 30-day follow up phone call. The characteristics of the eligible patients were that nearly a quarter of them (24.2%) were at least 75 years of age and 51.5% of them were women. The most common vascular risk of the group was hypertension (50.9%) and diabetes (19.5%), and 26.5% of the participants had active cancer. The most common surgeries that participants were undergoing were major orthopedic surgery (20.4%) and major general surgery (20.3%), and low-risk surgeries (39.4%).

The 30-day mortality rate was 1.9%; which amounted to 282 deaths with a 95% confidence interval and range of 1.7–2.1%. Over a quarter of patients (26.6%) died after hospital discharge; the median time from discharge to death was 11.0 days, and the interquartile range (IQR) was 4.0–15.0 days. Urgent or emergency surgery was the strongest preoperative predictor of 30-day mortality with an aHR of 4.62 and a 95% confidence interval between 3.57–5.98 days. The VISION group then used the minimum *P*-value within a multivariable approach to determine that the peak TnT threshold values of 0.02 ng/mL, 0.03 ng/mL, and 0.30 ng/mL were independently associated with 30-day mortality. The strongest independent predictors of 30-day mortality were a peak TnT value of 0.03–0.29 ng/mL (aHR, 5.00; 95% CI, 3.72–6.76) and 0.30 ng/mL or greater (aHR, 10.48; 95% CI, 6.25–16.62). Also, the VISION group distinguishes that independent predictive factors identified in their model possibly explain the majority of the deaths that occurred (the total population attributable risk was 89.0%; 95% CI, 85.3–92.4) since the predicted relevant peak TnT values had the largest population attributable risk (41.8%). Patients with TnT values that were independently associated with mortality in peak TnT measurement to death demonstrated the median times of 0.02 ng/mL (13.5 days; IQR, 8.5–20 days); 0.03–0.29 ng/mL (9.0 days; IQR, 3.5–16 days); and 0.30 ng/mL or greater (6.5 days; IQR, 1.5–15 days), $P = 0.01$. Overall, within the 282 patient population who had died within 30-days post-surgery, their respective health centers reported a vascular cause of death in 127 patients (45%) and a nonvascular cause of death in 155 patients (55.0%). VISION reported that the TnT thresholds that independently predicted 30-day mortality were not noticeably different for vascular or nonvascular mortality.

The VISION study was able to strongly associate the peak fourth-generation measurement of TnT within the first 3 days after noncardiac surgery with 30-day mortality. VISION's data suggests that 1 in 25 patients with a peak TnT measurement of 0.02 ng/mL, 1 in 11 patients with a peak TnT measurement of 0.03–0.29 ng/mL, and 1 in 6 patients with a peak TnT measurement of at least 0.30 ng/mL will die within 30 days of surgery. The VISION group reveals efficacy behind monitoring postoperative elevated TnT measurements to enhance risk stratification after noncardiac surgery.

Importantly, Devereaux demonstrated that 13.5% of patients having TJA had elevated postoperative troponin the risk of 1/7 type 2 nonischemic postoperative elevated troponin and cardiac complications was the same and we showed that risk could be avoided by cardiac anatomical assessment (OSCARs)of the patient 30 days before surgery. That is if this risk is type 2 myocardial ischemia not caused by coronary artery disease but caused by an imbalance between myocardial supply and demand as seen with HTN 68.1%, PAF 32.4%, CHF 53.5%, chronic kidney disease 39.6%, PE/DVT 5.3%, and other common causes [6].

That is if this risk is type 2 myocardial ischemia not caused by coronary artery disease but caused by an imbalance between myocardial supply and demand as seen with HTN 68.1%, DM 41.1%, PAF 32.4%, CHF 53.5%, chronic kidney disease 39.6%, PE/DVT 5.3%, and other common causes.

9.1 Results

Cardiovascular studies of elective TJA patients referred for preoperative evaluation showed:

- Ninety eight percent of people had at least one CV abnormality
- Seventy five percent had HTN with half requiring additional treatment because of LVH
- Fifteen percent total patients had diabetes

- Eleven percent had PAF and when stopping the anti-coagulation treatment, patients continued anti-arrhythmic therapy with sips of water before and after surgery, resulting in no PAF
- Of 33 patients with aortic dilatation, one had 52 mm 5% rupture rate AAA with endovascular repair then scheduled knee surgery.
- Three patients were found to have PE, cancelled surgery, and were under treatment.
- Several patients did not have surgical clearance by cardiologists due to graft occlusion but were rescheduled by our team because occluded grafts went to lesions that were not significant.

Our data compared to type 2 myocardial ischemia: HTN 68.1%, DM 41.1%, PAF 32.4%, CHF 53.5%, chronic kidney disease 39.6%, PE/DVT 5.3%, and other common causes.

Our complications postoperatively: ZERO Mortality

1. A patient whom we failed to treat for new HTN/LVH, RCRI low-risk mortality, OSCARs high-risk complications developed uncontrolled HTN and congestive heart failure and hospitalized an extra.
2. The asymptomatic patient, RCRI low mortality, OSCARs high-risk complications, with a complex coronary plaque ulcer on CCTA predicting an MI which occurred 24 h after surgery and resulted in angioplasty/stenting without heart damage with $10,000 cost savings.
3. A 68-year-old female RCRI low mortality, OSCARs high-risk complications readmitted 50 days post-op for chronic AF with a slow ventricular response.
4. A gentleman with SVT (200 bpm) prevented during THA but recurring 180 days post-op with syncope with readmission for radiofrequency ablation.

9.2 Conclusions

99% had uncomplicated TJA. OSCARs, based on pre-op imaging, reclassifies TJA patients as higher than RCRI score resulting in more aggressive perioperative management a prevention of PAF, hypertensive crisis with CHF, LVH, HTN, ruptured AA, and hypotension in AS. MI was predicted and treated based on plaque composition and morphology without heart or replaced joint damage. 99% of patients with cardiovascular image-guided disease-specific treatment did not have cardiovascular complications (one without treatment died) and could have had uncomplicated outpatient surgery. Continuation of our multihospital study using OSCARs by our Core Laboratory is recommended for acquiring a larger data set.

Don't forget! Three main points to take away:

1. Cardiovascular disease is now the leading cause of the most frequent postoperative non-orthopedic TJA complications especially in those >65 year old Cardiovascular +98% in patients.

2. Believed to be random, but by reducible OSCARs this risk is predictable: low EF, LVH >13, 24-hr BP/HTN, CVA/TIA, PAF, AAA/TAA, CAD/MI/plaque ulcer, PE/DVT, AS, General anesthesia or not regional; miscellaneous: rarer conditions.
3. Patients at reducible OSCARs risk can be recognized and treated for 30 days with predictable reduction of post-op cardiovascular complications allowing patients >65 year old to not have complications in the hospital, or readmissions, and to have orthopedic surgery without cardiac complications as an outpatient as well as extend longevity.

References

1. Sandoval Y, Jaffe AS. Using high sensitivity cardiac troponin T for acute cardiac care. Am J Med. 2017;130(12):1358–65.
2. Roche Diagnostics. Roche Elecsys cardiac Troponin T-high sensitive. https://diagnostics.roche.com/us/en/products/params/elecsys-troponin-t-high-sensitive-tnt-hs.html.
3. Rogers JK, et al. Effect of rosuvastatin on repeat heart failure hospitalizations: the CORONA trial (controlled Rosuvastatin multinational trial in heart failure). JACC Heart Fail. 2014;2(3):289–97.
4. Gravning J, et al. Prognostic effect of high-sensitive troponin T assessment in elderly patients with chronic heart failure results from the CORONA trial. Circ Heart Fail. 2014;7(1):96–103.
5. VISION Study Investigators, Devereaux PJ, et al. Association between postoperative troponin levels and 30-day mortality among patients undergoing noncardiac surgery. JAMA. 2012;307(21):2295–304.
6. Tripathi B, et al. Characteristics and outcomes of patients admitted with type 2 myocardial infarction. Am J Cardiol. 2021;157:33–41.

Palliation of Pain Secondary to Degenerative Joint Disease in the Inoperable Patient Population

10

Emilio Valdes

Abstract

The field of pain medicine has been expanding over the course of the last 20–30 years to meet the demands of a variety of different patient populations that suffer from diverse complex pain conditions. This chapter will offer medical providers a closer insight into the most current interventional pain procedures available for treating peripheral joint disease. The different approaches mentioned here will serve as a guide to establish the most appropriate pain management treatment plan for their patients. This chapter is unique in that it focuses on a specific subset of patients that are suffering from peripheral joint-related pain, who cannot be offered surgical intervention secondary to their medical comorbidities.

Keywords

Palliation · Palliative · Anesthesia · Pain · Degenerative joint disease (DJD) Peripheral nerve stimulation (PNS)

10.1 Case Presentation

A 78-year-old woman with a past medical history significant for atrial fibrillation on anticoagulation with Xarelto, insulin-dependent diabetes mellitus, hypertension, chronic kidney disease, morbid obesity, presents as a new patient to our outpatient chronic pain management practice. The patient suffers from chronic right shoulder, right hip, and bilateral knee pain. She has severe medial greater than lateral osteoarthritis affecting her right knee, this being her chief pain complaint. The patient has

E. Valdes (✉)
William Jennings Bryan Dorn VA Medical Center, Columbia, SC, USA

E. E. Harrison, N. H. Ho (eds.), *Managing Cardiovascular Risk In Elective Total Joint Arthroplasty*, https://doi.org/10.1007/978-3-031-26415-3_10

been denied surgical intervention until she can be medically optimized. What interventional techniques can be provided for this patient?

Although joint pain can be due to acute injury, trauma, or connective tissue disease (i.e., rheumatoid arthritis), in the overwhelming majority of patients it is a result of osteoarthritis. According to the CDC, it is projected that approximately 67 million individuals in the United States will suffer from arthritis by 2025 [1].

A multidisciplinary approach should always be taken when addressing any chronic pain condition; interventional pain physicians, pain psychologists, physiatrists, physical/occupational therapists, and neurologists are among the most common. It is beyond the scope and practicality of this chapter to describe all treatment options available for joint-related pain. Instead, it will focus on the interventional pain modalities that are currently available to target shoulder, hip, and knee pain. More specifically, we will address the following interventional techniques: diagnostic/therapeutic peripheral nerve blocks, radiofrequency ablation of peripheral nerves, and peripheral nerve stimulation.

10.2 Peripheral Nerve Blocks

Peripheral nerve blocks are usually performed under ultrasound-guidance and accomplished by utilizing solely a local anesthetic (i.e., lidocaine, bupivacaine), or a combination of local anesthetic and steroid (i.e., triamcinolone acetate, dexamethasone). If analgesia is accomplished from a peripheral nerve block, it typically only provides short-term pain relief and often has to be repeated every several weeks to months. This becomes a dilemma, since repetitive administration of steroids can lead to increased risk of infection, poor glycemic control, and further advancement of degenerative joint disease. The aforementioned negative sequelae from the repetitive administration of steroids has led interventional pain physicians to mainly perform peripheral nerve blocks for diagnostic purposes. If peripheral nerve blockade is confirmed to provide the patient with significant pain reduction, the use of radiofrequency ablation, and/or peripheral nerve stimulation can be offered to the patient with the goal of longer lasting analgesia.

10.3 Radiofrequency (RF) Treatment

Radiofrequency treatment, also known as radiofrequency ablation (RFA) or radiofrequency neurotomy, is a treatment that consists of the application of a high-frequency current by a needle to specific anatomic structures. Radiofrequency current heats the tissue surrounding the tip of the needle, thus producing a lesion. In interventional pain procedures, these compact lesions result in selective denervation. The size of the lesion depends on the temperature of the tip of the electrode, and tip temperature depends on the amount of power delivered. Other factors that influence lesion size include heat, type of tissue, and/or injection of steroid following completion of lesioning.

The radiofrequency probe is a simple electrode structure that generates radiofrequency energy when an electric current is passed through. These radiofrequency probes generate thermal energy in the surrounding tissue via ionic heating. Friction resulting from ions (Na^+, K^+, and Cl^-) moving generate heat, thus producing thermal destruction of the nerves. Neural tissue begins to denature or degrade at 43 °C.

Radiofrequency ablation treatments can be further classified into conventional, cooled, and pulsed. In conventional (traditional) RFA, a target temperature of 80–90 °C for 90 s is the goal. This will result in desiccation and charring of the tissues immediately adjacent to the probe because these tissues are absorbing the highest concentration of energy. Once these tissues become charred, they behave as an insulator that prevents any further energy to be moved beyond the charred tissue, which limits the size of the lesions created when conventional RFA is implemented. Due to these effects, conventional RFA lesions are elliptically shaped, as the charring follows the shape of the exposed electrode.

Cooled radiofrequency probes were developed in order to overcome the charring insulating effects that is associated with conventional RFA probes. In cooled radiofrequency probes, cooled water is circulated through the probe tip to maintain lower temperatures at the tissue-tip surface. The circulated cooled water carries the heat away from the tissue-tip interface, which in turn will diminish the desiccation and subsequent charring of adjacent tissues. As a result, cooled RFA has the ability to deliver more energy to the surrounding tissues, creating a larger area where ionic heating can take place. In cooled RFA, the tip temperature is set at 60 °C; however, research has demonstrated that the measured temperature beyond the tissue-tip interface reaches 80 °C. Where conventional RFA lesions are elliptical in shape, lesions produced by cooled RFA are spherical and larger. This affords the interventionist to reduce the likelihood of missing the target nerve. In addition to painful osteoarthritis of the knee, cooled radiofrequency ablation has also demonstrated durable clinical benefit in spinal indications such as discogenic pain and sacroiliac joint-related pain.

Pulsed radiofrequency ablation is a non-ablative alternative to conventional and cooled RFA. Pulsed RFA is delivered in short bursts, two times per second, followed by a quiet phase in which no current is applied. In comparison to conventional RFA (80–90 °C) and cooled RFA (60 °C), the goal temperature of pulsed RFA is set not to exceed 42 °C. As previously mentioned, neural tissue begins to degrade at approximately 43 °C. This is an important concept to understand because there are instances where cooled or conventional RFA cannot be utilized due to the increased risk of producing motor weakness or paralysis. In these clinical scenarios, the interventional pain physician may decide to utilize pulsed RFA. Since pulsed RFA does not result in destructive lesions, it is thought to produce analgesia via the creation of an electrical field and enhancement of descending modulatory systems. In effect, neuromodulation, which is defined as the alteration of nerve activity of the targeted nerve, theoretically takes place following pulsed RFA. Pulsed RFA has been used in the treatment of peripheral neuropathies, arthrogenic pain, painful trigger points, radiculopathy, and many other chronic pain syndromes. Even though there is significant anecdotal evidence that favors the use of pulsed RFA for the use of pain relief without nervous tissue destruction, there is a lack of randomized controlled trials (RCTs) supporting its efficacy. Further research in the clinical and biological effects of pulsed RFA involving well-designed, randomized controlled clinical trials with large sample sizes and long-term follow-up is required, in order to determine the therapeutic effect and safety of this treatment modality.

10.4 Peripheral Nerve Stimulation

Peripheral nerve stimulation (PNS) applies an electrical current to the peripheral nerves to relieve pain. Peripheral nerve stimulation was introduced by Wall and Sweet as well as others in the mid-1960s [2]. Patient selection is the most challenging and important step in the decision to offer neurostimulation. In order for a patient to be considered an appropriate candidate to undergo a trial with neurostimulation, the following criteria should be met: (1) the diagnosis is amenable to this therapy, (2) conservative therapy has failed to provide the patient with any significant pain relief, and (3) significant psychological issues have been ruled out.

With traditional peripheral nerve stimulators, patients will undergo a 5–8 day trial, which involves placement of a percutaneous electrical lead at the selected target. The percutaneous electrical lead is attached to an external battery during the trial period. During this period, the patient is encouraged to be as active as possible in their usual environment. At the end of the trial period, the percutaneous electrical lead is removed and the patient is asked a series of questions. Most interventional pain physicians consider a 50% or more pain reduction as a good indication of a successful trial. Besides the degree of pain reduction, other important factors to consider are change in activity level and medication intake. A combination of pain relief, increased activity level, and decreased medication intake indicates a favorable trial. If the previously mentioned factors are achieved during the trial period, the patient and interventional pain physician should have a discussion regarding proceeding with permanent implantation.

A permanent peripheral nerve stimulator usually comprises three parts: (1) electrodes or leads, (2) implantable pulse generators (IPGs) or the battery, and (3) the charging and programming systems. Not all PNS systems require permanent implantation. The SPRINT PNS System, by SPR Therapeutics, offers short-term, 60-day treatment which does not require permanent implantation [3]. This system has been studied extensively for low back pain, shoulder pain, post-amputation pain, and chronic and acute postoperative pain, working by selectively targeting peripheral nerve fibers. Recent clinical evidence has demonstrated significant reductions in pain often persisting well beyond the end of treatment following up to 60-day treatments, outcomes which have not previously been observed with conventional permanently implanted systems. One proposed mechanism of action is that by activating selective large diameter afferent fibers, reconditioning of maladaptive central nervous system changes associated with chronic pain occurs to induce a prolonged reduction in pain, thus avoiding a permanent implant.

The SPRINT PNS system includes the following:

1. Pulse generator: Worn on the skin to deliver gentle pulses to the nerve. Powered by a rechargeable battery.
2. Microlead: Coiled 300-micron lead is designed to allow fibrotic ingrowth to reduce migration and infection risk.
3. Hand-held remote: User-friendly design allows patients to easily adjust stimulation levels.

The SPRINT MicroLead is implanted and then removed after treatment for up to 60 days.

10.5 Shoulder Pain

The etiology of shoulder pain is diverse and can include pathologies arising from the glenohumeral joint, acromioclavicular joint, sternoclavicular joint, rotator cuff, and musculo-connective tissues of the shoulder girdle. In clinical practice, it is not uncommon to frequently encounter patients suffering from more than one of these pathologies simultaneously. The innervation of the shoulder itself is mainly by the suprascapular nerve and axillary nerve.

These two nerves are important targets in the treatment of chronic shoulder pain. The suprascapular nerve is considered to be one of the most important nerves in the shoulder region. The suprascapular nerve contains motor fibers to the supraspinatus and infraspinatus muscle, along with a major part of sensory fibers from the shoulder joint. The axillary nerve may be stimulated to improve lateral shoulder pain and motor functional abnormalities, while the suprascapular nerve may be stimulated to improve glenohumeral joint pain and motor pathology of the supra- and infraspinatus muscles. The suprascapular nerve can be modulated in the suprascapular notch above the scapular spine to target pain arising from the shoulder joint or from below the notch coming in from a lateral to medial approach [4]. Similarly, the axillary nerve can be modulated by placing a PNS electrode near the nerve either at the quadrangular space or at the surgical neck of the affected shoulder where the nerve and circumflex humeral artery are visualized [5]. Research in shoulder pain is a topic of critical interest and data is improving for both post stroke and degenerative shoulder disease [6].

10.5.1 Clinical Scenario

A patient with chronic right shoulder pain secondary to osteoarthritis of the glenohumeral and acromioclavicular joints who has failed conservative management, including intra-articular steroid injections, has been denied surgical intervention secondary to their underlying medical comorbidities. What options may be offered to this patient by the interventional pain physician?

This patient can be offered an ultrasound-guided right suprascapular nerve block as an interventional pain modality. This will provide the interventional pain physician with additional information such as the percentage in pain reduction achieved, duration of analgesia obtained following the block, changes in sleep quality, and changes in physical activity levels. Some patients with chronic shoulder pain may require targeting of both the suprascapular and axillary nerves in order to obtain significant pain relief. However, given that 70% of the afferent input travels via the suprascapular nerve, providing sensory input from the scapula, acromioclavicular joint, and posterior and superior shoulder joint, its blockade usually provides a patient with a noticeable improvement in pain. If the patient is simultaneously suffering from pathologies affecting the anterior aspect of the shoulder, an axillary nerve block may need to be simultaneously supplemented.

The patient undergoes a right suprascapular nerve block and returns to the pain clinic approximately 2 weeks later. He reports an 80% reduction of his shoulder pain and reported being able to sleep much more comfortably. However, these effects gradually diminished over the following few days and his pain intensity has returned to baseline. What other procedures can be offered to this patient?

Unfortunately, this scenario is frequently encountered. Although there are exceptions where patients respond to peripheral nerve blocks for an extended period of time, the analgesia obtained from most peripheral nerve blocks will diminish in a short period of time, usually within 15–72 h, if not in a much shorter period of time. Factors that may produce longer lasting analgesia following a peripheral nerve block include the type of local anesthetic utilized (lidocaine versus bupivacaine) and the addition of epinephrine and/or steroid to the local anesthetic solution. Nonetheless, peripheral nerve blocks should not be viewed as a long-lasting interventional pain modality. This is the reason why regional anesthesiologists implement peripheral nerve catheters with continuous infusion of local anesthetics following certain orthopedic interventions, thus maximizing longer lasting analgesia.

Now that the interventional pain physician knows this patient obtains significant analgesia from suprascapular nerve blockade, there are a few options that can be discussed. First, the patient can be offered repeat suprascapular nerve blocks as needed throughout the course of the year. Second, pulsed radiofrequency ablation of the suprascapular nerve can be discussed with the patient. As previously mentioned in this chapter, pulsed RFA is a non-ablative form of treatment that does not result in neural tissue destruction. The suprascapular nerve is a mixed motor/sensory nerve, therefore should not be treated with conventional or cooled radiofrequency ablation due to the risk of producing motor paralysis/weakness. As with any intervention, it is the responsibility of the interventional pain physician to discuss realistic expectations following this procedure. Further research is required to have a more accurate representation of the degree and duration of analgesia that is typically obtained following pulsed radiofrequency ablation of the suprascapular nerve. Even though this patient responded well to a suprascapular nerve block, this does not necessarily signify that the patient will respond similarly with pulsed RFA of the suprascapular nerve. Pulsed RFA, however, has the potential to produce longer lasting analgesia that can range anywhere from a few weeks up to 6 months. Finally, a third option that can be offered to this patient, is peripheral nerve stimulation targeting the suprascapular nerve. Peripheral nerve stimulation may include permanent implantable systems (assuming a successful PNS trial has been completed) versus a non-implantable PNS system.

10.6 Hip Pain

The sensory innervation of the hip joint capsule is complex and is divided into anterior and posterior components. The anteromedial aspect of the hip joint capsule is innervated by the articular branches of the obturator nerve. Additionally, the anterior hip joint capsule is innervated by sensory branches of the femoral nerve. The posterior segment of the hip joint capsule is innervated by articular branches of the sciatic nerve. Articular branches of the superior gluteal nerve have also been found to innervate the posterolateral segment of the hip joint capsule. Thus, effective neural blockade of the hip joint capsule must include the obturator nerve, femoral nerve, the sciatic nerve, and the superior gluteal nerve. Based on this information, one can deduce the challenges that may arise when trying to accomplish effective analgesia by means of diagnostic peripheral nerve blocks, radiofrequency ablation, and peripheral nerve stimulation.

Radiofrequency treatments for the sensory innervation of the hip joint (Fig. 10.1) have the potential to reduce pain secondary to degenerative conditions. Ongoing concerns remain regarding the anatomic targets, as well as quality, procedural aspects, and monitoring of outcomes in publications on this topic. Randomized controlled trials of high methodological quality are required to further elaborate the role of these interventions in this population [7].

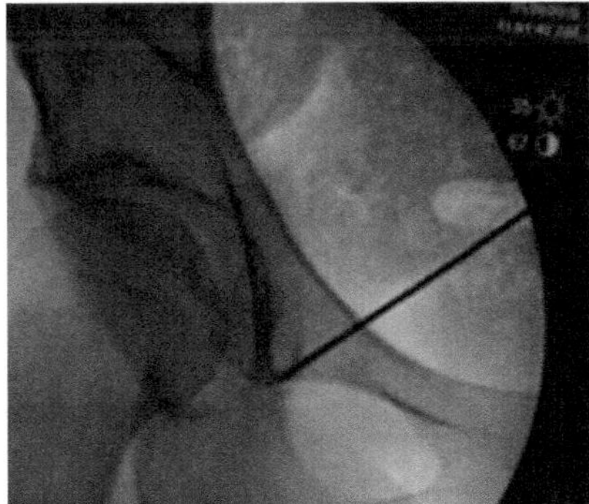

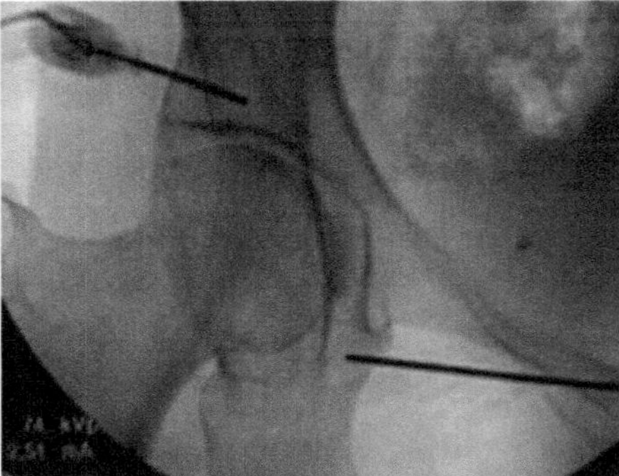

Fig. 10.1 Anteroposterior fluoroscopic imaging of the right hip during radiofrequency ablation of the lateral femoral and lateral obturator sensory branches using cooled radiofrequency electrodes

10.7 Knee Pain

Knee pain affects approximately 25% of adults, and its prevalence has increased almost 65% over the past 20 years, accounting for nearly four million primary care visits annually [8]. The prevalence of chronic knee pain secondary to osteoarthritis is 12% in individuals over 60 years of age. In addition to knee pain, osteoarthritis results in a decreased range of motion, muscle atrophy, and instability. Pain has the greatest impact on quality of life and is the leading catalyst for seeking medical attention.

Radiofrequency ablation (RFA) alleviates knee pain by targeting the intra-articular nerve endings originating from the genicular sensory nerve branches and/or periarticular branches of the saphenous nerve (Fig. 10.2). The genicular nerves have sensory contributions from the femoral, common perineal, saphenous, tibial, and obturator nerves. RFA of the genicular nerves most often involves targeting the superior lateral, superior medial, and inferior medial genicular nerves at their periosteal locations, precisely where the femoral and tibial shafts meet their epicondyles. The inferior lateral genicular nerve is not normally targeted due to its proximity to the common perineal nerve and subsequent risk of motor injury. However, if utilizing a pulsed radiofrequency technique, rather than conventional or cooled technique, the risk of possible motor injury is theoretically non-existent. Fluoroscopy is typically utilized to guide needle/probe placement; however, there are providers who utilize ultrasound-guidance for placement. Safe placement is confirmed by stimulation of the treatment area and observation of sensory nerve response without motor response before starting ablation.

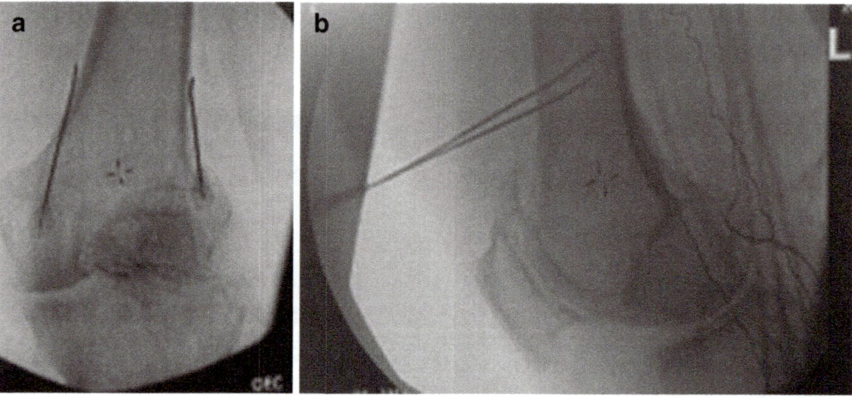

Fig. 10.2 Conventional radiofrequency ablative needles targeting the superomedial and superolateral genicular nerves on anteroposterior (**a**) and lateral (**b**) fluoroscopic views

10.8 Conclusion

Due to widespread advancements throughout the field of medicine, life expectancy has dramatically increased over the last few decades. Increased life expectancy has also led to an increased prevalence of age-related diseases such as coronary artery disease, cardiac arrhythmias, and valvular heart disease. Degenerative joint disease often accompanies patients suffering from these medical comorbidities. Many of these patients are denied surgical intervention as a treatment option of their peripheral joint disease due to an increased risk of mortality; therefore, other pain management options should be considered.

The field of interventional pain medicine has rapidly expanded throughout the last decades. There are now many different interventional pain modalities that have the potential to dramatically improve a patient's quality of life without exposing them to the increased risk of surgical intervention. In the overwhelming majority of these treatment options, infection risk is low and therapeutic anticoagulation may not even have to be discontinued.

The patient in the case presentation at the beginning of this chapter had a multitude of pain complaints; however, her right knee pain was causing her the most discomfort. One possible approach to this patient would be to offer her diagnostic genicular nerve blocks, which if proved efficacious, may be followed by performance of radiofrequency ablation of the right genicular nerves. Yet another approach may involve temporary versus permanent stimulation of the femoral nerve. If either of these procedures result in significant pain relief, it may allow her to engage in physical therapy or home exercise programs, which in turn could lead to avoidance of further musculoskeletal deconditioning and assist the patient in weight loss.

Furthermore, it is important to manage the expectations of patients in chronic pain. One important reason that may lead a patient to express dissatisfaction prior to and following a procedure is miscommunication. It is impossible to predict how much, if any pain relief, can be accomplished from any interventional pain treatment. Similarly, it is impossible to predict the duration of analgesia that a patient may experience following a successful procedure. Responses are variable, and this information should be effectively communicated to every patient.

This chapter has shed some light on some of the most common pain management scenarios as well as their treatment options. Regardless of your medical specialty, we are all encountering a more complex patient population. The most effective means of providing optimal care is to have a better understanding of our respective fields, a better understanding of medical pathologies, and having a better relationship with our patients.

References

1. CDC. Arthritis-related statistics. https://www.cdc.gov/arthritis/data_statistics/arthritis-related-stats.htm.
2. Benzon HT, Raja S, Liu SS, Fishman SM, Cohen SP. Essentials of pain medicine. 4th ed. New York, NY: Elsevier; 2018.

3. SPRINT PNS System. https://www.sprtherapeutics.com/.
4. Gofeld M, Agur A. Peripheral nerve stimulation for chronic shoulder pain: a proof of concept anatomy study. Neuromodulation. 2018;21(3):284–9.
5. Wilson RD, Bennett ME, et al. Fully implantable peripheral nerve stimulation for hemiplegic shoulder pain: a multi-site case series with two-year follow-up. Neuromodulation. 2018;21(3):290–5.
6. Mansfield JT, Desai MJ. Axillary peripheral nerve stimulation for chronic shoulder pain: a retrospective case series. Neuromodulation. 2020;23(6):812–8.
7. Bhatia A, Hoydonckx Y, et al. Radiofrequency procedures to relieve chronic hip pain: an evidence-based narrative review. Reg Anesth Pain Med. 2018;43(1):72–83.
8. Bunt CW, Jonas CE, Chang JG. Knee pain in adults and adolescents: the initial evaluation. Am Fam Physician. 2018;98(9):576–85.

Current and Future Trends in Orthopedics

11

Eric E. Harrison and David Elliot Teytelbaum

Abstract

History has shown that most of the techniques and equipment that surgeons are trained on during residency look much different than those used at the end of his/her career. These changes range from the sizes of incisions made to the types of imaging obtained. The pathologies observed in orthopedics remain constant, but the ways in which they are managed are subject to change. Therefore, it is imperative that surgeons remain as malleable as possible as they move forward in their career. In this chapter, we will discuss current trends in orthopedics and what the future may have in store moving forward.

Keywords

Robotics · ROBODOC · Total Hip Arthroplasty(THA) · Osteoarthritis (OA) Computer-assisted orthopedic surgery (CAOS) · VAS pain score · WOMAc pain score · Canakinumab Anti-Inflammatory Thrombosis Outcomes Study (CANTOS) · Embryonic stem cells

E. E. Harrison
Board Chair International Cardio-Oncology Society, ICOS CEO PrivaCors Inc. Cardio-Orthopaedics®, Tampa, FL, USA

Department of Medicine, Morsani College of Medicine, Tampa, FL, USA

Joint Special Operations University, Tampa, FL, USA

D. E. Teytelbaum (✉)
Exercise Physiology, FSU, Tallahassee, FL, USA

FSU College of Medicine, Tallahassee, FL, USA
e-mail: dteytelbaum@foreonline.org

E. E. Harrison, N. H. Ho (eds.), *Managing Cardiovascular Risk In Elective Total Joint Arthroplasty*, https://doi.org/10.1007/978-3-031-26415-3_11

It is not the strongest of the species that survives, nor the most intelligent. It is the one who is most adaptable to change.—Charles Darwin.

11.1 Robotics

The first robotic system purposed for orthopedics was the ROBODOC system developed at the university of California-Davis from 1986 to 1992. The inception of the idea was first attributed to remedy the early pitfalls of the cementless total hip arthroplasty (THA) which was overwhelmed with failure due to lack of ingrowth of bone and pain which was attributed to poor fit and stability of the implant. The system is a computed tomography (CT)-based, computer-aided robotic milling device that allows accurate preparation of the femoral bone and anatomic placement of the femoral component in cementless THA. The first human subject, randomized trial was conducted in three hospitals from 1994 to 1998 and showed statistically improved fit, fill, and alignment when compared to manual THA, and there were no intra-operative fractures in the robotic-treated group. However, the early robotic surgeries where not without its own unique problems of increased surgery times and the dependent risks associated such as increased blood loss and time under anesthesia [1].

Computer-assisted orthopedic surgery (CAOS) is an umbrella term that refers to all kinds of computerized tools, robotic devices, and instrumentations utilized for orthopedic surgery. CAOS is still in its infancy with less than 5% of surgeons in the USA, Europe, and Asia using computer-assisted technologies routinely. CAOS can be utilized throughout all levels of patient care from preoperative planning with CT-based virtual images (e.g., hip anatomy and cup replacement) to intra-operative robotic cutting tools during knee arthroplasty. Despite the relatively limited use of CAOS among surgeons, research and development around CAOS is prolific. The ratio of patents to publications regarding CAOS technology in the field of knee arthroplasty has increased from 1:10 in 2004 to almost 1:3 in 2014. Lack of CAOS adoption has been attributed to problems with "ergonomics and economics." Regarding ergonomics, Zheng et al. wrote that one of the barriers to adoption of navigation comes from "intra-operative glitches, unreliable accuracy, frustration with intra-operative registration and line of sight issues." Despite multiple studies concluding CAOS being cost-effective relative to manual arthroplasty, economics remains a common reason attributed to lack of adoption. This sentiment revolves around the high capital cost of robotic system and is further compounded by the increased operating expenses associated with longer surgery times [2–7].

Total knee arthroplasty has emerged as one of the leading adopters of CAOS. Multiple studies have showed that robotic-assisted TKA is associated with improved accuracy of achieving the planned femoral and tibial implant positioning, joint line restoration, and limb alignment when compared to manual TKA [8–12]. Other studies have supported the increased accuracy but continue to find increased surgery times [13]. A prospective randomized study by Park and Lee highlighted a series of complications in early surgeries attributed to the learning curve of performing surgeries with robotic systems [14].

There is no doubt that CAOS and adjacent platforms will continue to play a larger role in the future of orthopedics. What cannot be determined is to what degree this technology will undertake the roles of the surgeon or if it will ultimately serve as just another tool for the surgeon to utilize.

11.2 Stem Cells

Stem cell therapy can be described as the proverbial "wild west" of the orthopedic field. Commonly used types include embryonic stem cells, mesenchymal stem cells (derived from bone marrow, brain, liver, retina, pancreas, amnionic fluid, umbilical cord, and placenta), bone marrow stromal cells, and many others [15]. Due to their multilineage differentiation potential, mesenchymal stem cells were selected early on to be the focus of ongoing research and clinical trials [16]. Mesenchymal stem cells are able to differentiate into several different types of cells such as osteoblasts, chondrocytes, or adipocytes [17]. As mentioned above, mesenchymal stem cells can be derived from various sources but two specific sources, bone marrow and adipose tissue, have been the focus of research and development [18, 19].

Two recent meta-analyses identified seven and nine articles with 256 and 584 patients, respectively, that focused on mesenchymal-derived (bone marrow and adipose tissue) stem cell injections for the treatment of osteoarthritis. They found that mesenchymal stem cell injections significantly reduce VAS and WOMAc pain scores and reported little to no complications. The authors concluded that stem cell injections are safe and at the very least, show strong promise but require more research [20, 21].

Matteo et al. performed a systematic review and meta-analysis aiming to compare the effectiveness of bone marrow-derived mesenchymal stem cells versus adipose tissue-derived mesenchymal cells. They found 23 studies that matched their criteria, 10 examining bone marrow derivative cells, and 13 examining adipose-derived cells. They concluded that due to the lack of high quality studies and different protocols, it would be impossible to make any definite conclusions regarding the effectiveness of either source. However, they did conclude that there is currently no evidence to support either bone marrow or adipose tissue as a superior source of mesenchymal stem cells [22].

Ivan Martin who is the lead scientists at the university of Basel and his colleagues have been working on harvesting nasal chondrocytes and using them to grow new cartilage in the knee for the past 15 years. The lab obviously had to have a proof of concept and started with in vitro studies, then on to mice, followed by sheep, and finally two patients who have been followed for 2 years and so far, have not needed joint replacement. To harvest the cells, a small biopsy is taken of the nasal septum. These cells are then developed in a lab and loaded onto a sponge made of collagen to allow the nasal cells to colonize the sponge and develop new tissue. After 4 weeks, these cells are injected into the patient's knee joint. Martin claims that further clinical trials with a larger number of patients are required, but he is very hopeful [23].

11.3 Immunologic Drugs

Osteoarthritis (OA) is one of the most common diagnoses in the USA with approximately 10% of men and 13% of women over the age of 60 being effected [24]. Treatment for OA involves conservative treatment such as NSAIDs, physical therapy, and steroid injections or surgical treatment with a joint replacement. OA is coined a degenerative disease because it decompensates over time getting worse and worse. While the conservative treatments mentioned early may buy the patient some time before needing surgery, they do not alter the actual pathology of the disease. The pathophysiology of OA involves a cascade of inflammatory markers including interleukin-1B, IL-6, and tumor necrosis factor 6 (TNF-6). These markers then trigger proteins which are catabolic to bone and cartilage such as matrix metalloproteinase, ADAMTS5, and MAP kinases [25]. One marker in particularly, C-reactive protein (CRP) is very closely related to inflammation and painful osteoarthritis. Because CRP productions is triggered by IL-1B, IL-1 inhibitors such as Canakinumab have recently been of interest as a possible treatment for OA [25, 26].

Until recently, the studies that have looked at IL-1 inhibitors have proven to be unfruitful with no significance found in pain reduction scores between the experimental and control group. The initial spark of interest originated from an in vitro study where researchers found that canakinumab caused increased proteoglycan and reduced nitric oxide synthesis in human chondrocytes, effects that have been theorized to reduce cartilage breakdown [27]. These results had little to no clinical significance, until the CANTOS study. CANTOS (Canakinumab Anti-Inflammatory Thrombosis Outcomes Study) was a study that was initially looking at IL-1 inhibitors (Canakinumab) as a secondary prevention of cardiovascular disease. 10,061 patients with a medical history of previous myocardial infarction and a CRP level of 2 mg/L or greater received one of three different doses (50, 150, and 300 mg) of Canakinumab or placebo. Patients in the treatment group proved to have less infarctions, but the increased rate of infection nulled any mortality benefit. However, researchers presented a secondary analysis of OA data and found that combined incidence rates of total hip and knee replacements were 40–47% lower in the treatment group. It took 1 year for these results to be apparent. Importantly, the results remained significant when the subjects with a history of crystalline or inflammatory arthritis were excluded. These findings have drawn the attention of the orthopedic community only time will tell if they show to be a viable option for patients.

The field of orthopedics is cited yearly as one of the highest revenue generating sources for hospitals [28]. This makes the field very active regarding research and development of new products/procedures. While most of the field-changing innovations are out of the clinical orthpedic's hands, one can always keep an open and curious mind. Just as we accept and welcome change in every aspect of our life, such as the technology we use or the way we travel; physicians should meet change in their field with an open mind, and of course, a healthy degree of skepticism.

References

1. Bargar WL. Robots in orthopaedic surgery: past, present, and future. Clin Orthop Relat Res. 2007;463:31–6.
2. Picard F, et al. Computer assisted orthopaedic surgery: past, present and future. Med Eng Phys. 2019;72:55–65.
3. Zheng G, Nolte LP. Computer-assisted Orthopedic surgery: current state 642 and future perspective. Front Surg. 2015;2:66. https://doi.org/10.3389/fsurg.2015.00066.
4. Clement ND, Deehan DJ, Patton JT. Robot-assisted unicompartmental knee arthroplasty for patients with isolated medial compartment osteoarthritis is cost-effective: a markov decision analysis. Bone Joint J. 2019;101(9):1063–70.
5. Picard F, Clarke J, Gregori A, Deep K. Computer assisted knee replacement 812 surgery: is the movement mainstream? Orthop Muscular Syst. 2014;3(2) https://doi.org/10.4172/2161-0533.1000153.
6. Bäthis H, Perlick L, Tingart M, Lüring C, Zurakowski D, Grifka J. Alignment in 854 total knee arthroplasty. A comparison of computer-assisted surgery with the 855 conventional technique. J Bone Joint Surg. 2004;86(5):682–7.
7. Kayani B, Haddad FS. Robotic total knee arthroplasty: clinical outcomes and directions for future research. Bone Joint Res. 2019;8(10):438–42.
8. Song EK, Seon JK, Yim JH, Netravali NA, Bargar WL. Robotic-assisted TKA reduces postoperative alignment outliers and improves gap balance compared to conventional TKA. Clin Orthop Relat Res. 2013;471:118–26.
9. Moon YW, Ha CW, Do KH, et al. Comparison of robot-assisted and conventional total knee arthroplasty: a controlled cadaver study using multiparameter quantitative three-dimensional CT assessment of alignment. Comput Aided Surg. 2012;17:86–95.
10. Song EK, Seon JK, Park SJ, et al. Simultaneous bilateral total knee arthroplasty with robotic and conventional techniques: a prospective, randomized study. Knee Surg Sports Traumatol Arthrosc. 2011;19:1069–76.
11. Bellemans J, Vandenneucker H, Vanlauwe J. Robot-assisted total knee arthroplasty. Clin Orthop Relat Res. 2007;464:111–6.
12. Hampp EL, Chughtai M, Scholl LY, et al. Robotic-arm assisted total knee arthroplasty demonstrated greater accuracy and precision to plan compared with manual techniques. J Knee Surg. 2019;32:239–50.
13. Karthik K, et al. Robotic surgery in trauma and orthopaedics: a systematic review. Bone Joint J. 2015;97(3):292–9.
14. Park SE, Lee CT. Comparison of robotic-assisted and conventional manual implantation of a primary total knee arthroplasty. J Arthroplast. 2007;22:1054–9.
15. Kalamegam G, et al. A comprehensive review of stem cells for cartilage regeneration in osteoarthritis. Adv Exp Med Biol. 2018;1089:23–36.
16. Ballini A, et al. "Mesenchymal stem cells as promoters, enhancers, and playmakers of the translational regenerative medicine." Stem Cells Int 2017; 2017: 3292810.
17. Caplan AI. Adult mesenchymal stem cells for tissue engineering versus regenerative medicine. J Cell Physiol. 2007;213(2):341–7.
18. Wu L, et al. Regeneration of articular cartilage by adipose tissue derived mesenchymal stem cells: perspectives from stem cell biology and molecular medicine. J Cell Physiol. 2013;228(5):938–44.
19. Filardo G, et al. Mesenchymal stem cells for the treatment of cartilage lesions: from preclinical findings to clinical application in orthopaedics. Knee Surg Sports Traumatol Arthrosc. 2013;21(8):1717–29.
20. Wang J, et al. Mesenchymal stem cells-a promising strategy for treating knee osteoarthritis: a meta-analysis. Bone Joint Res. 2020;9(10):719–28.
21. Song Y, et al. Mesenchymal stem cells in knee osteoarthritis treatment: a systematic review and meta-analysis. J Orthop Translat. 2020;24:121–30.

22. Di Matteo B, et al. Minimally manipulated mesenchymal stem cells for the treatment of knee osteoarthritis: a systematic review of clinical evidence. Stem Cells Int. 2019;2019:1735242.
23. Cooney E. "Scientists engineer nasal cartilage cells to repair aching knees." www.statnews.com 9/1/2020. https://www.statnews.com/2021/09/01/engineered-nasal-cartilage-cells-knee-osteoarthritis/.
24. Zhang Y, Jordan JM. Epidemiology of osteoarthritis. Clin Geriatr Med. 2010;26(3):355–69.
25. Schieker M, et al. Effects of interleukin-1β inhibition on incident hip and knee replacement: exploratory analyses from a randomized, double-blind, placebo-controlled trial. Ann Intern Med. 2020;173(7):509–15.
26. Vincent TL. IL-1 in osteoarthritis: time for a critical review of the literature. F1000Res. 2019;8:F1000 Faculty Rev-934.
27. Cheleschi S, et al. Possible chondroprotective effect of canakinumab: an in vitro study on human osteoarthritic chondrocytes. Cytokine. 2015;71(2):165–72.
28. Moore C. "10 Physician specialties that drive the most revenue for hospitals." www.healthgrades.com 9/8/2020. https://www.healthgrades.com/explore/10-physician-specialties-that-drive-the-most-revenue-for-hospitals.

Index

E. E. Harrison, N. H. Ho (eds.), *Managing Cardiovascular Risk In Elective Total Joint Arthroplasty*, https://doi.org/10.1007/978-3-031-26415-3

GPSR Compliance

The European Union's (EU) General Product Safety Regulation (GPSR) is a set of rules that requires consumer products to be safe and our obligations to ensure this.

If you have any concerns about our products, you can contact us on ProductSafety@springernature.com

In case Publisher is established outside the EU, the EU authorized representative is:

Springer Nature Customer Service Center GmbH
Europaplatz 3
69115 Heidelberg, Germany

Batch number: 10370708

Printed by Printforce, the Netherlands